Beyond the Grip
of Craniosynostosis

Beyond the Grip of Craniosynostosis

*An Inside View of
Life Touched by the
Congenital Skull Deformity*

Kase D. Johnstun

Foreword by Katie Mae Garner

McFarland & Company, Inc., Publishers

Jefferson, North Carolina

LIBRARY OF CONGRESS CATALOGUING-IN-PUBLICATION DATA

Johnstun, Kase D., 1975–
    Beyond the grip of craniosynostosis : an inside view of life touched by
the congenital skull deformity / Kase D. Johnstun ; foreword by Katie
Mae Garner.
      p.   cm.
    Includes bibliographical references and index.

    ISBN 978-0-7864-7569-8 (softcover : acid free paper) ∞
    ISBN 978-1-4766-1771-8 (ebook)

    1. Johnstun, Kase D., 1975– 2. Craniosynostosis—Patients—
United States—Biography. I. Garner, Katie Mae. II. Title.
RJ482.C73J64 2015
618.92'097514—dc23   2014047886

BRITISH LIBRARY CATALOGUING DATA ARE AVAILABLE

On the cover: Kase D. Johnstun © Heather Bird Photography

Printed in the United States of America

*McFarland & Company, Inc., Publishers
  Box 611, Jefferson, North Carolina 28640
    www.mcfarlandpub.com*

For
my mom and dad

To
my wife and son

In rememberance of
Charlie Howard, a beautiful
boy the world lost too early

Acknowledgments

Thanks to, first, my mother and father, who made all the right decisions. I love you so much. Thank you to my wife, Mary, who is my best friend, biggest supporter, and the most patient woman I know—I am dull in your shine.

Thanks to those who were so willing to share to help others: Summer and Ryan Ehmann, Shelby Davidson, Robyn and Tommy Howard, Jamie and Stephen Hewitt, Kim and Wes Clark, Aimee and Jason DeVooght, Laurie and Joe Darnell, Calli and Dustin Rhoades, Tara and Shawn Pendleton, Jennifer McFarland, and to the brave man who shared his story with us but chose not to be named. You are all brave and your children are so lucky to have you, as I had my mom and dad.

Thank you to the doctors who opened their minds to me: Dr. Marion Walker, Dr. David Staffenberg, Dr. Nicole Jeffreys, and Dr. Jeffrey Fearon.

Thank you Katie Mae Garner and Cranio Kids, who first created a space for families to find one another.

Thanks to Amy Galm and CAPPS Kids for all the help along the way, to Cranio Care Bears for all they do for families.

To my mentors: thank you to Mike Magnuson, who taught me so much and always believed I could "swing with the big boys," to Chris Cokinos, who taught me how to weave research into prose, to Mikel Vause, who told me I needed to write, and to Jay Hart, who gave me my first love of the beauty of words.

Thanks to Sean Davis for his masterful artwork and for always picking up the phone when I call (figuratively and literally).

Thanks to Heather Bird for being not only a great photographer but also an amazing friend.

Thank you to my brother, Jake, for his friendship, his love, his support, and for dropping me on my head more than once while wrestling—Cranio Kids need to know they are no different from any other kids.

Table of Contents

Foreword

by Katie Mae Garner

"Craniosynostosis": it's a word that is painfully familiar to some and completely foreign to others. It became familiar to my husband and me on June 25, 2004, when our son Dillon was born with bicoronal and metopic craniosynostosis. My sister-in-law and her daughter were both born with bicoronal craniosynostosis, so it wasn't a completely foreign word, but it certainly wasn't one I expected to hear.

I've always been a researcher, fascinated with human science, so I set out on a quest to gain as much information as I could. I wanted to know exactly what this was, what caused it, and why my son's case was different from his aunt's and cousin's. My frantic search was fueled by fear, need for knowledge, and the hope that I would meet others in our situation. The only thing I found was that there were not nearly enough resources for families touched by this condition. There were some and they were good, but they were few. We felt alone. At that point, even before Dillon's first surgery, I had an idea and enlisted the help of some amazing friends to carry it through. I didn't want any family to ever feel alone again like Kase's mother did in 1975. The idea was Cranio Kids, and it officially went live in August of 2004.

In starting Cranio Kids, I anticipated a place where others would find information, comfort, and new friendships. I had no idea that I would be one of those who were comforted, and I'm thankful every day for the friendships and support I have gained through it. Believe it or not, a few beautiful things come out of this scary journey, and one of those things is the people who have come into our lives. It was through these people that I was able to meet Kase, a man who was born with craniosynotosis in 1975.

1

I was honored when Kase invited me to write this foreword. I was also extremely nervous; I wanted it to be perfect. Kase seems to have a gift for picking up on what people are feeling, as his communications to me immediately put me at ease. Reading the draft for this book further confirmed that not only is he gifted with understanding emotion; he's equally as gifted at putting those emotions into words and relaying them to the reader.

I knew when I read this it would likely cause some past emotions to surface. Within the first three pages, I could not put this book down. The powerful wording and raw emotion took me back deeper than I could have imagined. I felt as though I were right there next to the families he was interviewing and wanted nothing more than to be able to comfort and hold them. Rarely does an author write something that will hold my attention long enough to read a book in one sitting, but Kase did it. The medical history section was equally as fascinating to me, and it's that clear many, many hours were spent researching it. It contains information that I had not been able to find before all in one place, from archeological findings to the history of the first surgeries to correct the condition.

There are no two stories from families affected by craniosynostosis that will sound the same. All families affected by it have a condition in common, but their journeys are all different. If you're wondering if you should read this if you're not familiar with craniosynostosis, the answer is yes. Almost everyone has something that makes them feel different or insecure. Many parents have had children with life-altering diagnoses. Maybe you love someone who has been through something difficult and want to better understand what they're feeling. For all of you, the answer is yes. "Craniosynostosis" may be a foreign word to many, but fear, insecurity, joy, anger, and love are all universal.

Thank you, Kase, for this wonderful book and reminding me of how truly special and unique each journey is.

Katie Mae Garner grew up in a military household and moved from Illinois to Texas to Detroit before settling down with her husband, having two beautiful boys and starting Cranio Kids, a nonprofit organization dedicated to giving families of craniosynostosis a place of comfort, conversation and support. She is a full-time student studying physical therapy.

Preface

Some birth defects can be hidden while some cannot. Some will not affect the intelligence or growth of a child while some will. The birth defect craniosynostosis, the premature ossification of the cranial sutures, at times can be hidden and at times cannot be hidden. It can affect the growth of the brain of the child drastically, creating major developmental delays in the child and extreme physical abnormalities, while sometimes it may go unnoticed.

Will my child be slow developmentally? Will my child be made fun of because of his or her appearance? And, most important, should my child have major cranial surgery to release the fused suture? These are the questions whose answers parents want to know.

The answers are as varying as the types and severity of craniosynostosis. While most children born with craniosynostosis are born with the sagittal synostosis, many are not. While most born with craniosynostosis are given a clear diagnosis and treatment by competent medical teams, some children's conditions are dismissed, with doctors acting as if their parents are being paranoid about the shape of their child's head. For the most part, doctors know very little about why children are born with craniosynostosis. Recent studies have found genes related to the premature ossification of the sutures, but placement in the womb and certain pharmaceutical drugs have been linked to the premature ossification of the sutures as well.

But learning "why" a child is born with this birth defect does not tackle all the questions about what to do or what others have done when a child is or was born with craniosynostosis: that is what this book aims to do. The options, undeniably surgical in nature, are also varied, as the surgeons and medical texts interviewed and consulted, respectively, in the book nearly unanimously agree.

The pages that follow are not only a pilgrimage into the medical and sutural history of the cranium and the current surgical techniques to release the sutures but also a larger pilgrimage into the lives affected by the birth defect craniosynostosis. It is also a personal quest into how craniosynostosis, which I was born with in 1975, has changed my life and my relationship with my parents. There are silences that say too much, darkness in loss, scattered but fleeting personal revelations, and feelings of acceptance into something larger than myself: a group of children, 1 in 1,700, born with craniosynostosis. But, at the heart of this book there are families. Families who have had good luck with surgery. Families who have had multiple surgeries. And families who have, sadly, lost to craniosynostosis.

PART ONE: BEGINNINGS

1975

With craniosynostosis ... one of the most important things for them [parents] to understand, I think, from the beginning, is that the skull itself does not have the innate programming to grow. The skull is passive. The only reason that the skull grows is because the brain is growing under it, so the brain is really dictating the shape of our head. The brain is dictating even how our face grows, and what happens in craniosynostosis is that because one or more of the sutures have fused prematurely the skull is now dictating to the brain how it should grow. So it's now the reverse. The brain is being taken hostage by the skull, and so what we want to do, then, is release the hostage and allow the brain to resume normal control of the growth of the skull and the face.

—Dr. David Staffenberg, NYU Medical Center

I was born to make my mom cry. In 1975, fourteen hours before the start of the new year, before Dick Clark dropped the ball in New York City, and before everyone resolved to be a better person, the nurse who performed my Apgar test, minutes after my mom delivered me into this world, ran her hands over my head, looked toward my parents, and said, "Your baby is going to be a retard. He has no soft spots." She, without any other words, walked out of the delivery room to continue her work on New Year's Eve.

My mother bawled. My father held her. Her world, moments earlier filled with the joy of having a newborn son in her hands right before the new year—hope swimming in the time before the spring of life—fell apart. Exhausted from the birth process and devastated by the nurse's flippant regard for my mom's well-being, she fell limp on the delivery bed, only moving to eject the tears from her eyes.

My pediatrician, Dr. Way, came into the room to check up on the family. He had been my mom's pediatrician and took on my older brother and me as a favor to her. The favor didn't rise out of an elite social connection or a political tie between old families. My mom came from a rather poor family, but

Dr. Way, although he had a completely full patient list, accepted my brother and me with open arms, in short, out of kindness. And he was a kind man. Now, at thirty-eight years old, my memories of visits to his office are wrapped in warmth, something not all children can say. The walls and desks were painted warm pink, and fish, stenciled onto the glass separators between offices and waiting room, swam up and down. The rubber seats were soft and covered in plastic, and since I spent a lot of time in his office, I remember moving my hips back and forth just to annoy my mom, the squeaking of a small butt sliding across plastic cutting the air. Once seated on the paper that covered the bed in one of his patient rooms, I only remember smiles from the graying man, and in my mind I picture him to look like a young Andy Griffith. Earaches, the flu, the common cold, and headaches brought me to his office, unhappily walking in and sitting down, many times with a cold cloth wrapped around my head, dampening my then blond hair, but I only remember warmth when he came into the room.

"She said he is retarded," my mom said to Dr. Way when he walked in to see how the Apgar went and how the second addition to the Johnstun family was faring.

"Who said that?" he asked, his voice stern and angry, unlike the man I remember.

"Our nurse," my mom said.

"No, I want you to point her out to me," he said. His anger moved through the delivery room with a force that shook my mother and father, my father a man not easily shaken.

My mom pointed to a woman standing at the nurses' station.

"She's fired," Dr. Way said. "Do you want her fired? Because she's fired if you want it." His eyes grew with sincerity.

"I don't know if he ever fired her," my mom would tell me later, "but I don't remember saying yes."

Dr. Way ran his hands along my head and confirmed that I had no soft spots.

* * *

She screams and grunts and cries. She walks and breathes and squats. And with one final push, a child explodes onto this earth in a discolored bath of hope. The world's light shines into her newborn irises for the first time. Mom and dad look upon their miracle, their creation, and their new and immediate love. In a matter of a few painful hours, the future they had imagined for nine months has become present, present in the wiggling fingers and stretching larynx of a newborn. For a brief moment, they bask in the wonders of new life in the wheezy gasps of their child, they hug, and they stare into each other's eyes, exploring the depths of their bewilderment and wonder. Their future has arrived.

Every minute of every hour of every day, a baby is born. And before the doctor slaps the baby's bottom—more of a tradition now than a true medical necessity—parents worry. They worry about her little lungs. They worry about her fingers and toes. They worry about his eyes opening. They worry about all the limbs and appendages that make a baby beautiful. They hope the child's head looks round for the first photograph, because in developed countries healthy babies are expected and beautiful babies are desired.

A nurse takes the baby from his mother's arms, and like an engine she gives it a full, five-point inspection—an appearance, pulse, grimace, activity, respiration (Apgar) test. The baby cries in the corner while Mom and Dad wait for her first evaluation. With each criterion worth two points, the parents yearn for their son's first perfect ten—beautiful rosy skin, a pounding heartbeat, rich cries and coughs, movin' and shakin', and strong breaths. Most babies score between seven and ten points after one minute and their scores, if possible, increase at the five-minute test. They are cleaned and handed back to their mothers, ready to begin a new life full of ear infections and vomiting and the flu and the common cold, a new life full of the common ailments of children, ready to begin a life with undeniable possibilities, and their fathers' eyes light up with thoughts of future astronauts or presidents or software giants.

Nine months earlier, the child was a zygote, a constantly changing ball of cells, that spent a few days traveling through his mother's Fallopian tube before landing in her uterus, where he would spend the rest of his gestational life surviving, at first, solely on his mother's bloodstream. Religious or not, spiritual or not, the evolution and transformation of a ball of cells to a human baby that cries and spits and poops is nothing more than miraculous. This ball of thirty-two cells (the morula) divides into two—some cells create the embryo, while the others symbiotically create the shell that will protect and nourish the baby for months to come. During this embryonic stage, the baby is most susceptible to damage brought on by genetic miscalculations, as well as environmental intrusions—alcohol, X-rays, nutritional deficiencies, infection. During those first ten weeks of gestation, all of the major bodily organs are forming and they are mostly unprotected from random mutations at the cellular level.

The nurse lays the baby out on the table beneath a warming lamp and looks for any physical abnormalities. She places her finger in his mouth. She slides her hands through the baby's bottom and pushes a finger between the baby's toes and fingers. The palm of her hand and her fingertips caress the baby's head and read the scalp beneath the skin as if it were a braille tablet. She checks skin and lifts the eyelids. The father helps hold the child while the mother lies tired and crying and exposed only feet away. His hands shake with nervous energy built up from months of preparation and fear. His eyes follow the nurse's hands and his heart jumps on the slightest "humph," or "hmm," or "uh-huh" from the nurse's mouth. Was that a bad "humph"? Should I worry about that "uh-huh"? He asks himself these questions while the newborn is flipped and turned and wiped and swabbed.

Sometimes, something goes wrong—something that was not detected during the routine ultrasounds at twelve weeks and twenty-four weeks. While probing the baby's mouth, her finger might fall into the center of a deep cleft, ridged and rough and hollow; she might find a cavern where a cavern shouldn't be, and she may not have to probe at all before she discovers a gash of flesh that reaches from the inner mouth to the bottom of the nose. The nurse may run her hands down the lengths of the baby's arms and legs, measure the child's limbs, and find unusually short limbs and stunted bones. While sliding her fingers between the toes of the child, her finger might stop in a web of skin that prevents her finger from touching what should be the base of the toe or the finger. She might hesitate before announcing the Apgar score. Her eyes might close or look away for a moment before she turns to tell the worried parents that their child was born with a cleft palate or achondroplasia or webbed feet.

Birth defects are less rare than I would want to believe. Those caring nurses must turn to awaiting parents 3 times out of every 100 and tell them that something happened during the baby's development that caused a birth defect. More than 120,000 mothers in the United States drop their heads low and blame themselves for what had happened to their child. They scan their memory for mistakes along the way: Did I drink alcohol? Did I forget my vitamins? Did I not exercise enough? Did I gain too much weight? The guilt comes to them immediately, as they only blame themselves for their child's abnormality. But, for most, they shoulder guilt that is not theirs to carry. Even today, doctors know little as to why babies are born with birth defects. While scientists and doctors have made enormous leaps in identifying the genes that cause birth defects, they still do not know, for most babies, what created *those* genes. It is widely accepted in the medical community that 20 percent of birth defects are genetic, transferred to the child from one parent or both parents, and 10 percent are formed through environmental stress, drinking, and other substance abuse, so those poor mothers in the corners of the hospital rooms fall into the 90 percent of parents who had absolutely no control over what happened to their child at birth. But they will spend their life with an undeniable guilt that they somehow hurt their child just like my mother did when I was born with craniosynostosis—the premature hardening of sutures in the skull.

For some of us, the nurse may run her hand across the baby's skull and scalp and find that one or two or three of the soft areas of that scalp that allow the baby's brain to grow, the sutures, are no longer soft. She might check again because she thought she made a mistake or because she had examined twelve babies on her twelve-hour shift and she hopes that her mind may have drifted. On the second scan of the scalp, she concentrates on each nerve of her fingertips and slowly scans the head and sutures. Her fingertips move so slowly that she can feel every tiny hair on the newborn's head. She starts in the back, feeling the lambdoid suture first. It is pliable and soft, so she drags her fingers slightly forward to feel the triangular posterior fontanel, and it is soft and open. She breathes out, thinking that she had just made a mistake, but then as her fingers find the top angle of the posterior fontanel and begin to trace the sagittal suture, she feels nothing but hard, dense bone. The sagittal suture is fused. The baby's head will not be able to expand outward and therefore will disallow the child's brain to develop normally. She must alert the doctor. She must tell the parents. Something must happen to fix this child's skull. Many times, however, the nurse or pediatrician may not notice the hardened surface right after birth and the child will be sent home. His parents will watch the child's head, they will follow it with their hands, and they will notice that something is wrong, sometimes months, or even years, after his birth. Then it all begins.

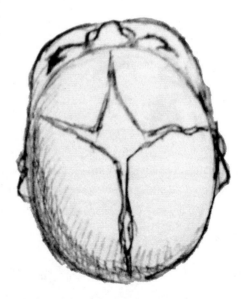

Babies' brains grow fast, likely doubling in size in the first nine months and tripling in size in the first

Normocephaly: the skull from the top view that shows all of the major sutures of the skull as they should be at birth, open. (courtesy of Sean Davis).

thirty-six months of their lives. Their skulls need to accommodate this growth, so they are born with fibrous hinges, or sutures, that allow the four bony parts of the skull (frontal, parietal, occipital, squamosal) to expand at the same rate as the brain, ensuring that the baby's brain grows as large as it needs to. When these sutures harden too early, the bony parts fuse together and don't allow the brain to expand at the rapid rate that is necessary for normal development. In the skull, like water flows over the least resistant path, the brain will grow into the areas of least resistance like waves that invade the caverns of a cave-laden shore. Depending on the suture or sutures that hardened too early, the skull would take a very specific shape, and the brain would have to fill it. There are four major types of craniosynostosis, with many subsets (more rare forms) of craniosynostosis, and each of them, it is believed, represents a different disease.

Most babies born with craniosynostosis suffer single suture sagittal synostosis (SAJ-ut-ul)—or scaphocephaly (SKAF-o-sef-a-lee). It is the most common diagnosis of the birth defect. When the sagittal suture fuses too early, the baby's brain cannot expand from side to side, and this forces the skull to bulge out over the child's brow and expand backward to a bony point. If the suture is not treated—if it is not released—the baby's head will look like a lopsided football, and a ridge of bone, like a mountain created by two tectonic plates slamming into each other, may rise off up from the baby's skull. My scar replaced my scaphocephaly. While this diagnosis is most common and most treatable, it is the one diagnosis that is prominent in males and exhibits a pattern of inheritance. Since babies' heads take many different shapes after birth, sagittal synostosis can go undiagnosed for months before it is discovered.

It's easiest to think of our skull bones like tectonic plates on our head. They are hard and imperfectly shaped. Our skull, like the earth, occupies a limited amount of space and our skull "plates" need buffers between them in order to move and shift and eventually settle. The premature hardening (premature ossification) of these buffers is most easily comparable to the slamming together of tectonic plates. In cases of metopic (mih-TOP-ick) synostosis—or trigonocephaly (try-GO-no-SEF-a-lee)—the ossification of the sutures creates a triangular forehead, eventually molding into a giant triangular skull above the nose, not to be confused with the presence of a metopic ridge, which does not necessarily denote metopic synostosis. The metopic suture runs from the bottom edge of the anterior fontanel to the top of the nose, and there is very little room for early ossification. The triangular bone structure that has risen off the forehead pulls the child's eyes inward toward the nose, and this inward pull can damage not only vision but also, obviously, brain development.

Unlike sagittal synostosis and metopic synostosis, doctors typically diagnose coronal or bicoronal (co-RO-nul)—anterior plagiocephaly [play-gee-o-SEF-a-lee] or brachycephaly [brak-a-SEF-a-lee]—synostosis soon after the baby's birth because of immediate misshapenness of the baby's brow. As the sagittal suture originates at the top of the cranium, the coronal sutures start, typically, on frontal left and right corners of the anterior fontanel and drop downward on the skull toward the ears and allow the forehead and frontal lobe to expand forward. If one or both of these sutures close prematurely, the baby's forehead will flatten out, his eye socket will rise and tilt (vertical dystopia [VUR-ti-kuhl dis-TOH-pee-uh]), the eyeball and eyelid will protrude (proptosis [prop-TOH-sis]), and his nose will move inward toward the affected side. If this type of craniosynostosis is not treated—besides having on onset chance at mental developmental delays—the child will suffer a number of vision problems for the rest of her life.

The fourth major type of craniosynostosis is the rarest. There are few cases diagnosed each year, and therefore it can be missed. Lambdoidal (lam-DOID-ul) synostosis, however, can be more subtle in its symptoms than the other three types of craniosynostosis, and since the lambdoid suture runs from the edge of the sagittal suture and downward like a V from the crown of the head to back of the head, it is commonly confused with flat head or just an abnormally shaped head, the commonly seen plagiocephaly—(plagiocephaly (play-gee-o-SEF-a-lee). There have been many misdiagnoses with this type of craniosynostosis that have led children with flattened heads to the operating room to have the sutures opened up when all they needed was physical therapy or a helmet to correct a common deformity. It's this misdiagnosis that makes an accurate estimate of cases difficult to obtain, but it is guessed to be 1 in 100,000 children, compared to that of sagittal craniosynostosis, which is estimated at 1 in 3,000 children. If this suture ossifies early, it does look like the common deformity of flat head, but many times the ear on the affected side will be pulled back and flattened. The pulling back of the ear, however, on the affected side should be an immediate indication that the child should receive a CT scan or diagnosis from a craniofacial specialist.

Most children born with craniosynostosis are lucky, though whether the word "lucky" could and should be used here is highly debatable, because nearly 85 percent of the babies are diagnosed with nonsyndromic craniosynostosis (NSC). NSC only ossifies the skull suture (or sutures) prematurely and leaves the rest of the skeletal system unmolested. Babies born with syndromic craniosynostosis, however, typically face a more devastating diagnosis than those who suffer the worst types of NSC. These early ossifications spread out from the skull and into the larger skeletal system, usually affecting the baby's limbs and extremities like the fingers and toes and are connected to syndromes such as Apert syndrome, Carpenter syndrome, Crouzon syndrome, Muenke syndrome, and Saethre-Chotzen syndrome. Children with these syndromes have a much smaller chance of leading a normal life than their NSC counterparts. Their feet and hands can be mitted. Their faces fail to develop fully. They have large, bulging eyes that pop forward from their underdeveloped faces. Even some of their larger bones, like their elbow joints and knee joints, ossify before full development and leave them immobile, but for the purpose of this work these syndromic cases will not be discussed in depth.

* * *

Dr. Way did not hesitate. He did not take the wait-and-see approach that tends to be the first approach of many pediatricians. He felt a hard skull where it should have been soft and sent us to a neurologist, Dr. Hauser. I would find nearly forty years later that the surgery had just barely become routine and the word "routine" would have had a very loose definition, somewhere between "less often" and "more often than a decade or two before."

My father wrings his hands and says that Dr. Hauser had a horrible bedside manner, that he was cold. He hurt my mother's feelings with his brashness, but my parents both agree that the second they talked to him they knew he was good at what he did. His frankness translated to confidence when we sat and talked about *their* story, and make no mistake, this was and never will be *my* story.

He told them how far surgery had come. He talked to them about the surgeons in Boston who had pioneered so many new and safe techniques. He filled them in on how and why babies had been lost in the past. He ran his hand down from one fontanel to the next and, with his nail, made a line in my scalp just off center and explained that he would make the incision there to avoid cutting an artery, a source of major blood loss and death in decades past. And he told them that I would be fine either way, with or without the surgery, but he also told them there was always a chance I could be "slow" and there was a much larger chance that I would not look like other children, that my head would not be able to grow outward on the left and right side but would continue to grow from the front to the back and bulge out above the ears.

They said yes. His words, his demeanor, his confidence pushed them that way. There were no support groups online, no Facebook page, and no one else to talk to, that they knew of, who had gone through the same thing. Sitting on an island alone, my parents said yes, long before they could have any certainties given to them.

They did it for me. They were scared of me being "slow"; they were scared of the future ridicule.

They said yes because their guts told them to say yes. My mother's intuition made the decision a nondecision.

"He has to be at least ten pounds for us to operate on him," Dr. Hauser told my parents. I was small at birth, barely topping the five pound, six ounce mark, so they set the date for my two-month birthday with the hopes that I would gain the necessary weight to handle the anesthesia.

"The day before you were to go into surgery, you hit the ten-pound mark," my mom said. "So we had to go through with it."

Those two months, however, did not sail along with just worrisome anticipation. One morning, I struggled for breath and gasped at the air around me, but my nasal passages, closed and underdeveloped, blocked the oxygen from reaching my lungs. As if someone had drawn a line around my head from the brow line, around and above my ears, right above the base of my neck and back around the ears on the other side to reach the brow line again, my skin had become a bright purple from the lack of oxygen to my brain.

The ER doctors shoved a breathing tube up my nose right before I passed out on the ER bed. I was born to make my mother cry.

"Will he be okay for surgery?" my mom asked the surgeon. He told her yes, but her mind latched on to another worry that she would carry with her into the hospital the morning that she and my father pulled into the parking lot of McKay-Dee Hospital in Ogden, Utah, and carried me in to check me in. Will he be able to breath? Will they watch to make sure his nasal passages are letting in air? Will that affect the outcome of the surgery? These questions, wrestling with all the other worries that had lived in her mind, pushed their way through and sat at the front of the line and led to one main question: Will he be breathing after this is all done?

They handed me over to the surgeons. The time between then and when the doctor came out to talk to my parents blurs, not only now in 2013, when my mother sits across from me and holds in tears, but even back then.

"I don't remember that time," she said. "I remember your dad holding me. He is so strong." She looks up at my father, who has decided to stand for the entirety of our talk. He leans over on our dining room chair and thinks about those days, doing his best to bring back those moments as vividly as he can for me, even though he'd probably rather be sitting next to me on the couch and talking about Kansas State football like we do, laughing and dropping in updates about work and life and anything else that crosses our minds, but he leans over the chair and tries to recall it all.

The search for details of what happened in the operating room that February in 1976 were nearly impossible to find. I walked into the medical records office of McKay-Dee and asked about the process of retrieving older medical records.

A woman, ready for her lunch, it seemed, pulling her brown sack out from beneath her desk, glared at me when I walked through the door with the "how could you bother me?" look smeared across her face.

"How far back?" she asked.

"Nineteen seventy-six," I answered.

She laughed at me, not a sympathetic chuckle but full-out laughter at my ignorant hope.

"We don't keep them that long. Wouldn't matter anyway. Most our records got burned in a fire years ago," she said, and then shooed me away by digging her hand into a bag of chips. I would return a couple months later after all of my efforts to find records in the two other local hospitals where Dr. Hauser had performed surgeries had dried up—the same response, though much nicer, but without the burning of records. The second lady I talked to at McKay-Dee was very kind, took my Social Security number, my name, and my parents' names. She took a few minutes trying to find me in the system, punching in different combinations of the information I had given her, and in those few minutes I had hope. I imagined her turning to me with a smile and then turning the monitor toward me and saying, "Here you are," and then letting me peruse the file while she ran my debit card through the machine to pay for the twenty or so pages that I needed to be printed out. But that didn't happen. Kindly, she looked back to me and told me that there was no surgical history for me. I left disappointed. More than that, I left devastated. Crazy thoughts ran through my mind like *Did I even have craniosynostosis?* and *Maybe I have been researching the wrong thing for two years* and *Am I a fraud?* I spun in this world of doubt and fear and insecurity about whom I was for months to follow and never shared my insecurities with anyone.

I'd be sitting at dinner, having a lovely time, and then, out of nowhere, doubt would enter my brain. I couldn't *prove* that I was born with craniosynostosis, and this ate at me. The ground beneath me felt shaky; my world felt imagined or contrived, like a bad novel where the main character has to be someone or something to make the ending right, but the reader doesn't believe the main character could do such a thing. My rug had been pulled out from under me; like pulling back the giant curtain and finding the Wizard of Oz, I felt scammed. I would even run my fingers down the long scar that could prove it all, but I still felt insecure without the proof that a piece of paper with my medical records could give me.

All this insecurity battled with the shame and guilt of not believing every word my parents had told me for nearly thirty years. They were there. They lived it. They heard the nurse say I would be retarded and one of best neurosurgeons in Utah tell them that there really was no option but to correct my synostosis. And by doubting them I felt shame, but I couldn't rid myself of all of these combating emotions and fears. I even contemplated writing something like "There is doubt about me even having craniosynostosis" in this book to clear my name from anyone who could say differently, and this too brought even more shame for doubting my mother who had held this inside her entire life—what a selfish person I had become to care more about my reputation than my mother's heart. All of this consumed me until I walked into Dr. Marion Walker's office at Primary Children's Hospital in Salt Lake City, Utah.

I hadn't planned on interviewing Dr. Walker until a good friend of mine, Dr. Nichole Jeffreys, talked to him about my book while they prepped for a surgery. She told me I had to talk to him, one of the best pediatric neurosurgeons in the country—she used the words "legendary" and "truly a pioneer." I didn't know what to expect when I walked into the conference room. I waited anxiously, even though this would be one of the last interviews I would conduct for the book.

Dr. Walker came to Utah in the mid-seventies and had performed hundreds, if not thousands, of surgeries to release the fused suture(s) brought about by their premature ossification. By the time I sat down with him, I had researched many, many different types of surgical techniques to correct synostosis, so I felt confident we could talk about them, and that was what I had hoped to gain from interview: an insight into the mind and experience of one the best and most respected surgeons in the country who not only had performed surgeries for the last forty years but also had performed surgeries using the techniques of most neurosurgeons, and I hoped to show him the one photo that showed my head before surgery and ask him to guess at my diagnosis—not surprisingly, very few photos were taken.

My mom has always said that she thought I was beautiful no matter what, and once when I told her that while I was digging for descriptions of my head pre-surgery and pushing my uncle to give me an honest description he told me my head looked like a football. My mom got angry as hell, saying that if someone ever said that to her she would have their heads. Once I convinced her that it was my doing, that I had pushed him to give me a description, she calmed down, as his intentions were only to help me, but I saw an anger in her eyes that I had rarely seen in my life.

I expected the interview to be strictly professional and sterile. I would be sitting across from a legend; I didn't want to show him the doubts and shame and insecurities I had been consumed by since I couldn't find a paper trail of proof for my craniosynostosis, but when Dr. Walker walked into the conference room, sat down, and folded his hands over his lap he filled the room with a calmness that I had not felt with any prior interview. He asked how I was, what I did for a living, if I had a family, and, finally, who the doctor was who performed surgery to release my sagittal suture.

"He did a good job," Dr. Walker said.

I had recently shaved my head for the first time in my life and shaved it again for this interview, so he could see the work of Dr. Hauser. I told Dr. Walker about his bedside manner and all he said was, "He was a hell of surgeon." Then he rubbed his hand over his head and smiled.

"I'll take that over niceties anytime," I said.

He laughed.

"Are you sure it was sagittal?" I asked. I turned so his eyes could follow my scar.

"Absolutely," he said. "That's the exact scar line for that suture. We couldn't get at the other sutures that way."

Why I questioned his sage knowledge I have no idea and I feel silly now as I recount the meeting, but I pulled up the photo that I had to have him look at before I left.

"What about this ridge?" I asked. "Could it have been metopic?"

"Nope. That's just your skull pushing forward. Happens all the time with sagittals."

Right then, I felt so selfish to push him to look at the photo, but that same peace swept back through the room.

"He did a great job with you," Dr. Walker said.

All that worry, that insecurity, fell away. All that had built up and made me feel like a fraud disappeared that moment. This man I had never met before had solidified the "me" that had been defined by my craniosynostosis. All that was left was the shame for doubting for even the slightest moment what my parents had told me.

I had hoped to be a professional with him, but something about him broke down my barriers, and by the time I left that day I had asked him all the little things that I never felt comfortable asking anyone else. He told me about the evolution of the surgeries. He filled me in on the introduction of plastic surgeons to the medical teams to correct the synostosis and how he believed they were a great addition. He shared his views on endoscopic surgeries and full cranial vault reconstructions, which I will share later in this book, and he told me how he believed my surgery was performed in 1976:

> Sagittal had been done for a long time. The worry early on was that it would grow back together. So they tried to do things so it wouldn't grow back together. They put solution on the dura, because the dura helps create the bone for growth. They would line little plastic strips along where we had taken the bone off. None of that worked. The bone regrew. So, over time, we learned that doing a wider craniectomy worked much better. With very small children, it's the shape of the brain that's gonna make the shape of the head, and your skull reshapes very quickly once you take off a wide strip for the sagittal suture. I've personally never been convinced that the Pi technique and the major reshaping have been necessary for sagittal. The strip craniectomy works very well and has worked for decades. I'm guessing that's exactly what he did with you, and he did it well. He was a good surgeon that your parents put their trust in.
>
> Parents come to us all the time. A pediatrician or someone has told them that there is going to be brain damage if they don't have the surgery. We've seen kids at five or six years old who come in and we haven't seen before. They are falling behind in school and suffering headaches. It just gets too tight in there. There's a lot of untreated sagittals walking around, so it's hard to predict if one thing leads to another, but for the baby, they're not going to have brain damage by next week. There's always going to be damage if it gets too tight, but there is no rush for surgery. I just prefer operating at six weeks for sagittal because the skull is so flexible, but other doctors wait longer, and there is no worry about that wait as far as the brain goes.

His hands fell back over his lap and he asked about my boy and our move back to Utah.

"Swimmingly" was the word Dr. Hauser used to describe my surgery when he walked out to greet my parents, but I don't think he would have used this image of a child floating in liquid if he could have predicted that moments later I would begin to lose blood like a sponge being wrung. The red liquid filled my bandages until they could no longer handle the thin, deep red liquid and let the blood seep out, dripping like that same sponge letting go of its last droplets of water. Too much blood was lost. At ten pounds, there was very little room for the large outward flowing of blood. The staff ran to the doctor and let him know what was happening. He ran to the nurses' station only to hear that blood for a transfusion had not been requested or that they had requested the wrong type.

"We could hear him yelling at the staff from your room. He yelled at them so loud. He was so mad," my mom said. But his anger, his words, and his yelling at the top of his lungs to get some blood to my room were just sounds in her periphery.

Blood had seeped from my bandages, and my chest caved in.

"You had this indentation in your chest. You struggled so hard to breathe," my dad said. "It was like someone had indented a quarter into your chest and your lungs pulled that quarter to your spine. That's how small your chest was, like your ribs touched your spine, trying to get air."

Over the years, I had heard about the surgery, about what the doctors told them, and even about how my head had turned purple from lack of oxygen a few weeks before my surgery, but I had never heard about the moment when I had lost too much blood, when my chest had sunken in, and when I had fallen into severe respiratory failure. This was the story that my mom had avoided telling me for years, the one that brought her to tears and ended conversations. I had always wondered where the shock came from and where her reasons to block it all out and leave it behind were spawned. And, during this talk, I had forced her to relive it, and the guilt of it all weighed heavier on me than coming face-to-face with my own mortality and the realization that I am lucky as hell to walk this earth—that would come later.

My chest had caved in. Her legs moved. Her body followed until she stood outside shivering and said good-bye to me.

"It's time to call your priest and your family," Dr. Hauser had told my parents—the priest for my last rites and my extended family to say good-bye.

"I felt like I wasn't me anymore," she said. "Like I was someone else watching me walk into the cold and stand there and cry." She stood like a ghost above herself, and her world didn't seem real anymore.

Across from me at the table, her tears finally came. It was the moment in my story that she felt like she had seen my last breath that brought her to tears thirty-eight years later, the moment in the story I had never heard.

"Your dad is so strong," she says through her tears. "Without him..." She trails off, and he finishes the story.

"As soon as the blood started entering your body, you came alive immediately," he says. And, across from me, my mom's tears start to dry.

"Sorry I got emotional," she says, as if she shouldn't have. "I guess this is why I repressed it all these years. Your dad is so strong." She laughs at herself and forgets her own strength.

Out of the Chutes

North of Denver in Mead, Colorado, a man yelled at me to slow my car from 20 miles an hour to 15 miles an hour as I circled the suburban block of Summer Ehmann's home, the home of my first interviewee and the co-founder of Cranio Care Bears, a nonprofit organization created to do one thing and one thing only: give comfort to mothers and fathers of children with craniosynostosis before, during, and after their child's corrective surgery.

Lost in thought, in nerves, and in exhaustion, after driving eight hours the night before from my home in Manhattan, Kansas, I had, according to the man on the street, put too much pedal to too much metal, so he waved at me, and with his palms pointed to the ground he moved them up and down, and just in case he thought I wouldn't understand the international wave for "slow down," he raised his hands in the air and flashed two full hands of fingers and then one full hand of fingers. Luckily, there was no one else on the road at the time, because I may have hit them with my car while counting out the number of fingers in the air.

I am always early. I'm one of those people. I get up early, so I can shower early, so I can worry about arriving on time for hours before leaving way too early to arrive way too early. It's not that I love being early. I just hate to be late.

I pulled my little black car to the side of the road on the other side of the cul-de-sac and fumbled through my leather briefcase for the digital voice recorder that I had just bought minutes before at Target and for my notebook—bought minutes before at the same Target—my pen, not bought at Target but stolen from the Days Inn where I had slept the night before. While I may always be early, I am rarely prepared.

The clock ticked on the dashboard, and at exactly 10:30 I grabbed my briefcase, shoved my hand into its exterior pocket one more time, and scanned the contents with my fingers to make sure that I had everything I needed. The brown, weathered briefcase and its interior contents weren't needed, but their presence in my left hand seemed scholarly and professional, so the bag came with me.

There was no real reason to be nervous; Summer had been beyond nice in our correspondence and had expressed true excitement about the project. Her e-mails ended with smiling emoticons and explanation points, the new punctuation of excitement and happiness, but the walk from the car to the door shoved blades of sharpened nerve pains in my stomach and rumbled my bowels, the lifelong sign that I was nervous as hell, but the knock on the door produced two tiny faces in the long windows that lined it, Summer's children, one of them, Brentley, a boy born with craniosynostosis. Their noses spread out wide against the glass, and their eyes stared up at me. I waved at them, but they just stared back.

On an unusually wet and windy day in the fall in the Mead, Colorado, area, a plastic swing that had been attached to the deck ceiling swung close enough to me that I raised my hand to shield my face, even though there was no real chance of getting hit. The hand raising to block the swing made me feel less awkward as I stood there with four eyes pinned on me.

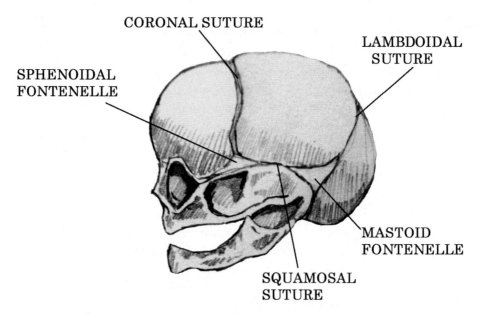

The profile view of the skull that shows the open sphenoid suture that was closed when Brentley was born (courtesy of Sean Davis).

Then, like every household with young children, Mom followed her kids to the door after finishing up any last bit of cleaning or straightening up before a stranger came to her home for the first time. I have seen my wife do it a million times and even hold me at the front door so she could shove one last toy back into place.

Summer opened the door with the same smile I had seen on her Web site photo. In the photo, she holds Brentley so tight that their faces seem like one. He is just a baby, maybe three months old. She smiles big but with what seems to be hesitance, and Brentley smiles too. This photo was taken pre-surgery, and Summer's hesitant smile is one of fear and confusion. Brentley's open-mouthed, no-teeth smile sits below two eyes that are not symmetrical. His right eye is wide and blue and beautiful like his mom's, but his left eye is nearly shut, like he's giving the camera a big cheesy wink. Above it, his forehead is slightly concave and pushes downward on his eye socket and cheek and the left side of his head slants downward from the crown. He grasps his mother's arm like any baby would, closing one to two fingers around the edge of her shoulder. While the world can see his misshapen head and eye in this photo, he is handsome and happy and loved.

At the door, little Brentley, along with his sister, peek out from behind the door. Like children do, they stare up at me and scan my face and clothes and eyes. I give them a quick "hello" and "good to meet you," and I do my best to not stare at Brentley's head. While 1 in between 1,700 and 2,000 children are born with cranio each year, the young boy in front of me, who hops with anticipation of someone new in his home, is the first person I have, knowingly, met who shared my birth defect. I give him a wink, and he runs away, his two-year-old attention span eventually winning out and pushing toward things that are much more exciting than the nearly forty-year-old man standing in the doorway.

"Hi, Kase," Summer says. Her voice is calm and welcoming and her hand-shake makes me feel welcome immediately. She is one of those people who make those of us who freeze up with nerves and shyness feel at ease, only confirming the feeling that I already knew her.

Within the previous month (September 2012), Cranio Care Bears had won the first Aveeno "Be An Active Natural," a grant given to a cause that positively impacts the world, so I had seen Summer on the Denver morning news and had seen that her hair had grown longer than it was in the photo with her and Brentley. I had watched all the videos on her Web site, and so when she opened the door and said hello, in my mind I already knew her. She did not know me, but in this social-media-connected world, where people spout out knowledge about your recent trip to Barcelona or your son's trip to Pumpkin Patch even though you've never met them, these moments have become common, and if I were to say at the moment, "I know all about you," it wouldn't have been weird at all.

On the way to her living room, Brentley and his sister zoomed by our legs, pushing cars and making toys fly, and Summer's husband, dressed in his Saturday work clothes, a sweatshirt and saggy, worn-in jeans, walked from the garage, where he had been tinkering and cleaning and working, and extended his hand.

With a firm handshake and a genuinely welcoming smile to match Summer's, he said, "Good to meet you. I'm glad you're here." Then, as if a passing ghost uncomfortable around the living, he walked away into the garage. I'd expected him to say more, to add to the interview, but as if previously decided, he would be on kid duty for the entirety of the interview, and to be honest, he did seem very happy to see me but not very motivated to talk about their experience, so, with a nod that said "see you later," Summer and I made our way to their couches and began to talk with no awkwardness or uncomfortable pauses, mainly because Summer was ready to tell her story.

On December 20, the night before Brentley's surgery, though only forty miles from Children's Hospital Colorado in Aurora, Summer and Ryan Ehmann packed up six-month-old Brentley, his skull pushing down on his eye and the left side of his skull lying flat against his face, and stayed in a hotel close to the hospital, leaving their daughter, Braylee, with Ryan's mom, who had flown in from Montana to watch over her during the next few days or weeks, the nearing future too volatile for the couple to easily predict their time away from home.

The family escaped the hotel room and wandered the aisles of the Bass Pro Shop, Brentley unknowing of what awaited him in the morning. Summer and Ryan did what they could and went where they could to spend time with their young son, alone, the night before his doctor would open up his skull and slice into the miniature suture, the frontal sphenoid suture, a very rare form of craniosynostosis where the miniature suture between the sphenoid bone and the occipital bone had fused so the orbit of his eye was stuck to the larger bones of his skull and could not grow.

They saw Santa there. It was Christmastime. But Santa's red coat and long white beard could not calm the Ehmanns, as anticipation hung above them throughout their night.

In the morning, they sat in the waiting room and played with toys and snapped photo after photo after photo. Summer wanted photos of Brentley as he was, knowing that he would never be the same again, and she wanted to remember the face of the boy she had loved since giving birth to him nearly six months earlier.

It was upon them. They moved from the waiting room to the pre-op room, and it was in the pre-op room at five in the morning where the sharp reality of the surgery took hold. In a few minutes the doctor would take Brentley away, and Summer and Ryan would not be able to see their son until post-op many hours later.

Ryan and Summer dressed Brentley in a little gown and gave him water and Pedialyte. The pre-op team washed his head with a sterile liquid, and when Brentley fell asleep in his mother's arms the room had become hopeful, stressful but hopeful, until the pre-op nurse began to list the all of the possible complications, although the possibility was minute, that could become reality because of the surgery. The realities were startling.

"Because of the blood transfusion, he could get AIDS," the pre-op nurse said in an emotionless tone, doing what she needed to do, what was required of her to say before any surgery that would require a blood transfusion.

"AIDS?" Summer screamed aloud in her head. "AIDS? I didn't know about this one. I need to talk to somebody now!" She was frightened.

"Also, since we will be operating around his eye, there is a chance he could go blind," the nurse said in the same monotone. "And he may not wake up from this surgery."

By this time, Summer had begun to laugh. The what-ifs began to pile up so high that her laughter reflex had taken over and she just wanted the what-if lady to leave, the extra weight of possible complications heaved on top of the already-known possible complications, the ones that Summer had built up strength to accept. It became too much. But with enough time, the what-ifs stopped, the lady left, and Summer whispered, "I don't ever want to see that lady again." It was a rational response from a freaked-out mother, and within minutes the anesthesiologist, neurosurgeon, and nurses had eased Summer's mind by answering every question that the what-ifs lady had raised.

"We're going to take care of your son as if he were our own," the neurosurgeon said.

Then the nurse took Brentley from his parents' arms. The white walls of the hospital surrounded the woman in blue who carried the little boy down the short hallway to the double doors of the operating room. The nurse's green surgical cap covered her hair and ears and neck, as if a faceless person had carried Brentley away, but sitting on her shoulder as she walked away Brentley's face bobbed up and down. He did not cry. And his little pacifier sat snugly in his mouth, a smile poking out from beneath it.

The nurse wrapped both arms around Brentley and wedged her clipboard with all of the baby's information beneath the blanket that was wrapped around him. She stopped briefly to push the button that opened the double doors in front of her, and they opened up wide—the yellow and black automatic door Caution sign slowly turning from broad side to thin side.

Ryan Ehmann is a man's man. He's a rodeo champion. YouTube is covered with videos of Ryan flying out of the chutes on top of a bareback horse. The horse beneath him jumps and turns and spins. It kicks and snarls and bucks. But Ryan spurs the horse, his body flails back and forth and forward and backward. Dirt flies into the air behind him and the crowd cheers until the eight-second horn screams into the air, and Ryan jumps into his dismount, landing hard and fast on his knees and back and feet. He walks with a limp, his body torn up from more than a decade of championship riding, and, even at forty years old he is lean and sinewy and muscular, a man who has probably never backed away from anything because of fear—most recently, he appeared on *Shark Tank* and walked away from the show with a deal and has become Cowboy Ryan, a national fitness icon, but when the nurse took Brentley away, Ryan's voice shook as he said, "Bye-bye, Brentley." Ryan's voice was timid and soft and fading. It cracked and barely broke through his lips. The man who had wrestled horses for decades struggled to get out words, and his worst fear walked away in front of him. His Brentley might not come back.

The nurse, to that point, had done her job. She took Brentley from his parents, did not look back at them, and headed toward the operating room. But, at the last second, before she turned the corner and disappeared, it looked as if she turned her face to the baby boy and gave him a kiss, and then, as she turned and as her profile became visible, she turned her head to his little ear, the one that slanted slightly downward, and whispered something to him. She looked to be comforting him. Then she was gone.

"That might be the last time I see my child," Summer said to herself. She looked at Ryan, who had shut off the camera he was holding, and he told her that he felt the same way. When the rodeo cowboy began to cry, her strength left her, and they cried together as they walked toward the waiting room doors and began what would be the longest morning of their lives.

Sometimes we never know who will step into our lives and help us through times that tear our souls from our insides and lay them out for everyone to see. In the waiting room during Brentley's surgery, the front desk lady, as Summer describes her, was that person, someone who, knowing it or not, had the ability to dilute the tears during painful moments. The desk lady, unlike the what-ifs lady, told jokes and made Ryan and Summer laugh throughout the four-and-a-half-hour surgery. Between hourly doctor visits to relay updates, the desk lady helped the Ehmanns feel a little bit of comfort and relaxation and hope. Laughter has a way of cutting through fear and pain and worry, and the desk lady gave them laughter, enough for Summer to think of her a year and a half later and smile and clasp her hands over her heart and smile again.

The hourly phone calls from the doctor talked about blood transfusions and incisions and progress until the final call came that alerted the Ehmanns to the completion of the surgery. Brentley was okay. The surgeons said that it had gone as well as it could have, that they had to reconstruct his eye socket because it had become misshapen, and, most important, they had separated the bones of his skull that had been prematurely fused, releasing his skull to grow normally as Brentley grew up, eliminating the chance that his brain would follow his skull in misshapenness and creating a normal-shaped head for the young boy.

It was time to see their boy.

* * *

Six months earlier, in June 2010, Brentley was born. Within days, Summer's mom had begun to point out Brentley's lopsided head. It wasn't as if Summer and Ryan denied the lopsidedness of his head, but they had attributed it to the normal cone-headedness of newborns, and their pediatrician, during the first two months of checkups, believed it was the journey through the birth canal that caused Brentley's head to be misshapen too, so every time Summer's mom brought up Brentley's head and the way it slanted downward toward his eye, Summer dismissed her worries as worries that all grandmas have about their grandchildren. *He was fine.* The only thing Summer wanted to believe was her pediatrician's affirmation that Brentley's head was fine and that the slanting of it was from the birth.

"That's enough about his head," Summer told her mom over and over again for the first two months of Brentley's life. "Enough about his head. He's fine. It's just from the birth." But, in her heart, she knew that his head wasn't getting better over time, that his skull hadn't begun to round itself out, but, despite what her gut instinct told her, she wanted his head to be just fine.

At the two-month checkup, a nurse-practitioner, one they hadn't met yet, came in to perform the routine checkup. He looked down at Brentley. The tension between grandmother and mother grew within the room when Summer's mom asked, "What do you think about his head?"

Summer rolled her eyes back into her head, she gasped loudly with frustration and denial and said, "There's nothing wrong with his head. They already said nothing's wrong with him." Despite Summer's objection to the idea that something was wrong with him and despite her outward frustration with her mother for asking the same question that she had asked for the last two months, the nurse-practitioner took his hands and began to push on Brentley's skull, an action that did not make the two-month-old boy happy, and even though the boy whined and complained, the practitioner continued to push against the boy's skull until he scanned the entirety of Brentley's head. The man's face showed stress.

"I don't think his plates are moving," the man said. "It could be what they call craniosynostosis." A nurse-practitioner and a foster parent, the man explained to Summer that he had seen multiple children with craniosynostosis, including one who had complete ossification of all sutures, come through his home. He knew what he was talking about. As a foster parent, he had become very familiar with the birth defect and was able to not only correctly diagnose but also explain it to Summer and her mom that day.

"I'm not really sure this is it. I can't really move the plates with my hand, but he could have coronal [craniosynostosis]," the man said. The shape of the eye, the downward pull of the skull, and the shifting of the ear made coronal a strong and more recognizable possibility.

The words that came out of the nurse-practitioner's mouth sounded like Swahili to Summer. She didn't understand what any of them meant, except for that they meant something was wrong with Brentley, and anger and resentment rose up inside of her. *Who is this guy? I want my regular pediatrician back,* Summer thought. All she felt was anger toward the man in front of her.

"Well, can we ask Dr. Quintana?" she asked. Her voice had a snarkiness, rudeness, in it that even now she remembers as uncharacteristic of herself. She didn't care.

"Of course," the nurse-practitioner said. Then he picked up Brentley and took him out of the room and into the hallway.

Summer, not wanting to be left out of the conversation, poked her head out of the room and into the hallway just in time to hear her regular pediatrician say, "I really don't think it's cranio. It really doesn't look like it."

I believe him. There's nothing wrong with my son. He's completely normal, my doctor said, so stop talking about it, ran through her mind. *That was that.* She clung to the hope that there was nothing wrong with Brentley, knowing that if she admitted something was wrong something would have to be done about it, knowing that if she let the possibility in she would have to accept it, figure it out, and live with the consequences.

Her curiosity won. At home that night, Summer held a piece of paper in her hand. The nurse-practitioner had written the words "coronal craniosyn-ostosis" on it at Summer's request. She placed the piece of paper next to her computer and did what we all do in this age of Google. She Googled cran-iosynostosis. What she found shocked her. Hurt her. Scared her to death. The images that popped up on the screen showed the children with engorged heads, with cleft palates, with arms and legs that had been fused straight at the joints, missing bones in faces, and eyeballs lifted or dropped below each other. The Internet, her Google search, scared the hell out of her, so when she lay down in bed that night the only images she saw were those of the children on her computer screen; the images of malformed children swirled around in her head, keeping her awake until the morning sunlight dropped and rose above the plains of western Colorado and fell into her window the next morning. As soon as the doctor's office opened, the receptionist received a call from Summer demanding to set up an appointment for a CT scan for Brentley.

She watched her baby slip beneath the massive machine to get his head scanned, his little body tied down to make sure he didn't move, his mother there to nurse him for comfort. "Horrific" was the only word Summer could think of when she talked about the memory of her son being made to lie still as the fluorescent light of the CT scan ran back and forth above his head.

"He doesn't have cranio," her doctor told her, words that only built up her denial that something was seriously wrong with Brentley's head. The boy's coronal suture was wide open, so her doctor believed it was positional plagio-cephaly, a flattened-head disorder caused by an infant lying on one part of his head for too long, creating a flat area on his head that is usually matched with the growth of little hair in that area, and that Summer should lay Brentley on the other side of his head for the next couple months so that the positional plagiocephaly would fix itself.

So that's exactly what she did. Religiously, she placed Brentley on his back when she put him down to sleep, placed wedges beneath his head to prevent him from rolling over onto the front side of his head where his skull had become flat, and watched him with the diligence only given to a mother, but in the back of her head none of this made sense to her. Her little boy had always slept on his back, but the flatness of his skull was on his front. When the doctor tried to explain how this could happen, while she wanted to believe it, something ate at her every day. Then, two months after she had begun to place Brentley on his back to sleep, she noticed that flat part of his head had gotten flatter and his eye had closed more, because of the pressure of his skull pushing down on it.

At the four-month checkup, Brentley's head, even though he had been laid on his back for two months, hadn't gotten any better. When the pediatrician came in to talk with Summer and she expressed her concern, she hoped that he would tell her that a helmet, the common way to fix plagiocephaly, would be the most efficient way to fix her son's flattened head, knowing at that point, of course, that none of the invasive surgeries to fix craniosynostosis would be needed because the CT scan had ruled out that possibility because all of the major sutures were wide open. She hoped her doctor would wipe away her fears with the suggestion of a helmet that she imagined decorating with stickers and paint and drawings, a helmet that would mold her son's head back to normal, a helmet that confirmed the diagnosis of placiocephaly, not craniosynostosis.

The pediatrician did not brush off Summer's worries. He did not order a helmet. Instead, he became very concerned and left the room. Summer's mom, who had accompanied her that day, held back her tears to create a sense of calm, but Summer could not. In her mind she wondered where the helmet was, why the doctor wasn't measuring Brentley's head for a helmet, and why things weren't going the way she had expected them to go that day when she packed her things that morning.

When her pediatrician came back into the room, he did not have a helmet but a referral to a neurosurgeon at Children's Hospital Colorado.

Summer left that day without the reassurance that she had hoped for and with the thought that her pediatrician had referred her to the neurosurgery department at Children's because that was where they handed out the helmets, holding the thought at bay that the diagnosis could be much worse, while feeling a small sense of relief that no matter where the road took her and her family, someone was going to do something to fix the boy.

Summer's hope was dashed. In the neurosurgeon's office at Children's, the nurse-practitioner walked into the room, took a brief look at Brentley's head, and told the Ehmanns that he needed surgery because what she saw was an obvious case of craniosynostosis and he would need surgery to fix it.

"Wait, wait. We just came for a helmet. We've had a CT scan. No cranio. That's what it showed," Summer said to the friendly but curt nurse-practitioner who had given her the bad news.

"Cranio is not fixed with helmets. We don't normally do CT scans here to diagnose cranio, and I'm pretty sure he has cranio just by looking at him," the nurse-practitioner said.

"Well, I want to see the doctor," Summer said. She'd begun to lose control inside. Her rage at the inconsistencies between the diagnoses, at the use or disuse of the CT scan as a tool to diagnose, and the uncertainty that the nurse-practitioner had just given her made her head spin with all the dark, but natural, thoughts of a mother: *What if I lose my son? Are we're going to have another baby to replace him? What will his funeral be like?*

The neurosurgeon, along with the plastic surgeon, traced Brentley's head with their hands, took notes, and confirmed what the nurse had said: Brentley had craniosynostosis and needed surgery to correct it.

Summer had dreamed of a helmet on her son. She imagined decorating it with stickers and art and asking people to sign it and putting it on his shelf for him to look at when he grew up. For Summer, the helmet was a simple fix. It was a gift. The doctors' diagnosis crushed that dream, and when the nurse came in to schedule surgery not only did Summer begin to bawl, but she also let in a depression that would stay with her for months, and those thoughts of her son's death, of his funeral, and of his possible replacement flooded her, even though she did whatever she could to keep them out. She knew they were horrible and combated them with logic and love: *You can't replace a child. Everything will be fine. I really don't feel this way.*

The Ehmanns left Children's in a haze of confusion and darkness. The CT scan showed no craniosynostosis, but the doctors said yes to the diagnosis. At two months, the Ehmanns' boy was normal, but at four months he was not. Two hours before, Summer had already decorated a helmet in her mind, but the Ehmanns left the hospital without a helmet to decorate.

The young family drove from downtown Denver where the man-made skyline blocked out the sun and headed north toward Mead, Colorado. The snow-covered Rockies to the west followed them home along Interstate 25. In the back of the car, Brentley and Braylee sat in their car seats, oblivious to what was happening in the front seat, their parents thinking about a surgery two months down the other side of the road.

At home, in front of her computer, Summer scanned the original CT scan from her pediatrician's office. The CT scan showed Brentley's skull. The thick part of the skull was light gray, nearly white, and the sutures, the open parts of the skull, were black like dark, thick canyons on a rounded plain. On the skull of a baby with craniosynostosis, one, or more, of the sutures will look as if it didn't exist—the dark void between the white plates of the skull is filled up with the same solid whiteness of the skull bones.

The open sutures fell from Brentley's diamond-shaped fontanel to the sides of his skull. Summer scrolled through the images until she found the image of Brentley's coronal suture, the suture the doctor had diagnosed as closed. But, there in front of her on the scan, Brentley's coronal suture that dropped from the fontanel down to the left side of his eye was as dark, black and open as the rest of his sutures. It was not fused. After she had been tossed around, back and forth between the negative diagnosis and positive diagnosis, the wide-open coronal suture in front of Summer put at the top of the roller-coaster again, and she dropped down into the depths of pure confusion, anger, and fear—again. In less than two months' time, doctors planned to open up her son's head. They planned to take him away from her and fix a coronal suture that, to her, looked wide open, and they planned to operate on a baby who did not need to be operated on.

Within moments, she had Children's on the phone.

"Someone needs to dig up that CT scan," she said to the nurse-practitioner. Summer made them dig and look closely. She was correct. The coronal suture was open, but the doctor, having scanned the CT, found that the tiny, tiny suture next to the boy's eye was closed, and although the suture was so little, the effect of it being closed would be just as damaging as if it were a large suture. His skull was fixed to the bones around his eye like a freighter held to a dry shoreline by an anchor; nothing else could move like it should.

* * *

The walk to the boy's bed in the pediatric intensive care unit (PICU) took less than twenty seconds. Summer rushed forward while Ryan hung back a bit and said aloud, "Is that him, that's him?" Beeps from machines and swishes from hospital booties were the only sounds that filled the PICU besides Ryan's excited but shaky voice.

Summer's short, dark hair covered her face from the side. She carried a camera in her hands to capture the first moment she would see Brentley, but as she got to the side of the crib she dropped the camera into one hand and placed the other on the crib's railing. Plastic liners surround the crib, and he lay with his eyes open—both of them open. In the middle of his skull, a tube stuck out and blood flowed through it. The surgery had left an incision that zigzagged from his left ear to the crown of his head, and stitches held two sides of his scalp together. At the end of the incision, near the ear and closet to the ossified suture, the incision looked deeper and the blood looked thicker. But he was awake.

Summer clasped her hand against her chest, and Ryan arrived by her side. A nurse stood across from them on the other side of the crib. Summer's lips pursed, and she tried to hold back her tears.

"My baby," she said. Her voice was high but quiet. With her words came her tears, and like her, when Ryan looked down and said hello to his "little buddy" the tears came, as if the mouth was a conduit to the heart and words a recognition of the reality, placing them in that moment of post-surgery, a moment they had looked forward to since the first diagnosis of craniosynostosis four months earlier.

Summer's hand left her chest and pointed to Brentley. "Why is he shaking?" she asked.

"He's probably ready for a drink," the nurse responded.

Ryan continued to talk to his "little buddy" until he said exactly what Summer was thinking: "He looks beautiful."

* * *

I stood in their doorway, ready to leave, excited about our conversation, and the three of us made small talk about where I could find a good beer and lunch. Some ideas were thrown my way, and they discussed the different options. The mood had become even more relaxed and friendly. The credits for *Toy Story 2* rolled on the TV above us, and the children continued to pull toys from their toy box, chances are, returning the house back to the condition they would prefer it to be in, toys readily accessible in all places of the living room. I saw it in Ryan's eyes then. He didn't think I was a bother. He just didn't want to relive the moments that had brought the rodeo king to his knees.

Brentley, mid-conversation, running and jumping and playing, ran too close to the coffee table, tripped on what I could only see to be carpet, fell forward, and hit his head on the edge. Summer, mid-sentence, hit the floor and had Brentley in her arms before the first of many tears flew from his eyes.

"Augh, he's a tough little guy. He'll be fine. At least you know his head can take a lot of beating," I said with my entire foot shoved in my stupid mouth. Just like always, I tried to defuse the situation and make it more comfortable for me to live in, and, like always, I would have to live with the stupidity of the words that fell from my mouth.

As if taking him back into the womb, Summer cuddled his entire two-year-old body into her torso, pushing his hair out of the way and scanning his head. Bright red and covered with tears, he pushed out cries, and with one swipe of her hand across his head his zigzagged scar, the one she had shown me earlier, became visible.

It's as if I had forgotten that he had craniosynostosis, his childhood playfulness and excitement and normalcy placing that fact far in the back of my thick skull, as if I'd forgotten that he, a little more than a year earlier, had his skull sawed open, fixed, and then cinched back together again and had months of recovery covered with bandages and helmets and his mother's worry. His parents had to deal with this, and the handsome young man lay in front of them crying after slamming his head against the coffee table.

Before Summer said anything to me, the boy crying in her arms, I could see in her face all the pain and fear that she had gone through during diagnosis, surgery, and recovery. When Brentley stopped crying, Summer gathered herself and with the same genuine kindness she forgave me and said, "I think your mom would probably understand." Summer didn't say anything else, but I knew what she meant—once your child goes through something like that, you can never stop the worry.

Kinship

It is just this year, at the age of thirty-eight, that I feel a true kinship with a very large group of people outside of my immediate family. I walked into homes, met people at coffee shops, sat in the sun at park benches, and sat in doctors' offices. I took photos with children in New York City, in Seattle, and in Kansas City. I saw hundreds of photos and CT scans, all placed down in front of me by the shaking hands of mothers and fathers who were not only willing to share their stories but also hoping their story could help just one other family who had gone through or might have to go through the struggles and disappointments and fears, as well as the victories, they had to go through.

When I began this, I was worried that all the stories would sound the same. There would be a diagnosis. There would be worry and fear about an upcoming surgery. There would be the day at the hospital when the child was taken into the operating room, and then there would be recovery of skulls and families. But I was wrong, more wrong than I could have imagined. Every family I talked to had gone through something different. They had different doctors. They had good surgeries and bad surgeries, one surgery and multiple surgeries, "swimmingly" good surgeries and botched surgeries. Some had families who supported them and some had families who told them to just "buck up" and stop complaining and whining about their child.

All the stories were different, and each of them, I hope, will touch another family like theirs. At thirty-eight years old, I feel a kinship to a much larger family, to children all over the world who were born with a closed suture or sutures that will define them, and I feel blessed to be one of the 1 in 1,700 children who are born with craniosynostosis.

PART TWO: THE REARVIEW MIRROR

Sutures

Surgical repair, resculpting, and reconstruction of the cranial sutures sits on top of a pin in the sands of prehistoric and recorded history, as these procedures to release the cranial sutures are still in their seminal phase, but the medical history and neurosurgical study of cranial sutures can be dipped far into the sands of recorded time. Hippocrates, known as the father of Western medicine, along with his students, wrote many treatises that reinvented the world of medicine in ancient Greece, discrediting the idea that injuries and illnesses came naturally and were not distributed by angry gods.

Hippocrates and his students, most influentially in *The Hippocrates Treatise* on head trauma written in 400 BC, described and mapped the morphology (the shape, structure, and patterns) of the skull and the cranial sutures. The treatise examines the skull in great detail. It looks at the structure of the normal human skull, its thickness, and its shape. The book also illustrates the importance of the connective tissue in the body and focuses on the connective tissue in the cranium—he describes where the bone tissue becomes thicker and thinner, softer and harder. The treatise also describes an in-depth analysis of the differences in the softer and harder connective areas in children and adults, defining craniology and setting the groundwork for neurosurgeons and craniofacial surgeons who would come more than two thousand years later. He also believed that the sutured areas of the skull were more susceptible to injury and that if someone was hit on the suture lines he would suffer more damage than if he was hit anywhere else on the head. Within the treatise, a skull without sutures is clearly defined. It developed with an odd shape because of its lack of sutures, and that skull would be our first medically examined skull that dealt with the relationship between sutures and skulls' shapes.

While Hippocrates dug medicine out of the dirt of philosophy and mythology by creating a methodology of listening to patients, examining patients, and understanding the medical history of patients—defining Western medical structures we understand today—there was very little he could do surgically in ancient Greece to repair fused sutures or a traumatic injury to the skull, and during his time dissection of the human body was not permitted, so his studies were done through observation and diagnosis, not through opening the skin and looking inside. Most believe that after Hippocrates' death the medical advances of the ancient Greeks slowed drastically, the influencer of the movement no longer pushing the boundaries of medical discovery and diagnosis. His treatises, however, and the Hippocratic oath that doctors still repeat today live long after Hippocrates and his students examined the morphology of ancient Greeks, illustrated and charted them, and used them to seed future advances of craniology and neurology.

The knowledge of the pliability of the skull, however, and the use of this pliability to morph the head has been around for thousands of years in different areas of the world, across thousands of miles and oceans away from Hippocrates. Many cultures used head sculpting to elongate, flatten, and mold infants' heads by binding the infant's head between two pieces of wood as if the metopic and lambdoid sutures were simultaneously closed. They tied cloth around the head to create a very round shape. They did this, typically, starting at one month after birth and kept the binders or cloth in place until about six months of age, which matches the months in which doctors, today, typically watch the closures of sutures. They knew 200 years BC, and before that, that by constricting the natural growth of the human skull, and brain for that matter, at a young age the skull shape would remain that shape for the rest of the infant's life or at least grow in similar fashion. The concept of head sculpting was developed broadly across cultures and times, meaning that it was discovered, developed, and implemented many times and by many cultures without knowledge of other cultures' participation in

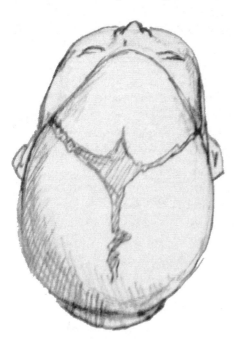

The skull with metopic synostosis (trigonocephaly) (courtesy of Sean Davis).

the ancient and not so ancient (as some cultures still sculpt infants' heads today) practice, dating back to more than 10,000 years BC and continuing until today. Hippocrates mentioned some and knew of some during his time, calling them the long-headed men. To name a few, there were the Huns, the Mayans, the Incans, some East Germanic tribes, and multiple Native American tribes, as well as some Australian tribes—eliminating the possibility that the practice started in one part of the world and was carried to other parts, as these distinct civilizations reinvented the practice of head morphology in different times and different places. The reasons for the morphology of the skull can only be speculated on and probably varied significantly across the globe, but the truth cannot be discounted: the knowledge of at least the purpose of the sutures, even if not a clear knowledge of the sutures themselves, has existed for tens of thousands of years.

The concept of natural morphology based on restricted suture growth, oxycephaly (noted to be the most serious of "-phaly" of craniosynostois), was first defined by Galen of Pergamon (AD 129–199). Galen of Pergamon is regarded even more highly than Hippocrates, as he was known for his unbiased look at medical discovery, and this lack of bias was apparent in his writing. Another benefit garnered by Galen came through his travels. Galen was able to dissect large animals such as gorillas, monkeys, and other large mammals similar to humans. While many of his writings were wrong because he attributed some animal anatomical knowledge to human anatomy, most of his writings and descriptions were unbelievably accurate. This accuracy leads most researchers to the belief that while Galen was in Egypt he had the chance, outside the watchful eyes of Greek society, to dissect humans. There are many stories of Galen saving kings and queens from, for instance, a common stomachache when current medicine called for drastic bloodlettings or even more severe treatment. Galen, like Hippocrates, prescribed natural healing methods such as diet, exercise, and rest. He was unequaled in his time, and it was he, most feel, through his dissection of large mammals (and perhaps humans), who discovered premature closing of the cranial sutures.

While Hippocrates used his hands and observations to analyze the sutures, Galen took it a step further and found open as well as prematurely closed sutures and observed and wrote about the first instance of oxycephaly, the shape of the head created by the closing of the lambdoid suture, and therefore, craniosynostosis. Also, following in the same vein as Hippocrates, Galen pushed back against the writings of the great Greek philosophers, mainly Aristotle, who believed that the brain functioned only in a supplementary or supportive role to the heart. Aristotle believed that the brain's function was one of an air condi-

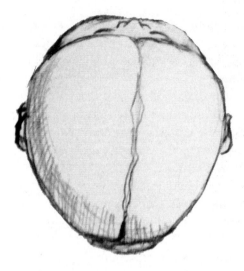

The skull with bilateral coronal synostosis (both coronal sutures closed at birth) (courtesy of Sean Davis).

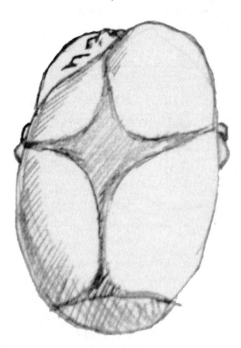

The skull with unilateral coronal synostosis (one of the coronal sutures closed) (courtesy of Sean Davis).

tioner for the heart as it pumped phlegm downward toward the heart and the phlegm cooled the beating mass in the chest. While the brain cannot survive without the heart, Galen's extensive study of the nervous system came in direct opposition to the teachings of the great philosopher and pushed Galen to promote the brain as the most important organ in the body, as it controls every activity in the body through the miles and miles of veinous highways. Most interestingly, Galen drew one very important conclusion: since the brain is the most important organ in the body and since the brain controls all functions in the body, if the brain is traumatized or compressed it will harmfully affect the body. It sounds as if Galen was the first physician not only to recognize the importance of the brain but also to recognize the importance of the brain having plenty of space to grow and work—he was hypothesizing about the problem of ICP (intracranial pressure) almost two thousand years ago and recognizing that ICP obstructed the brain's work and therefore the health of the individual. After Galen, most physicians in Western medicine used his writings as scripture until his writings were challenged hundreds of years later, although much of what he had written centuries earlier still lingers, with validity, in medical textbooks today, so what was described and written about before the start of Christianity has not been debunked.

Galen recognized that the shape of an infant's head and then an adult's head could be detrimentally affected by the pliable sutures and unsecured plates beneath the scalp and dura, but Andreas Vesalius, an anatomist during the Renaissance, found a lot of what Galenism taught to be incorrect. He had the opportunity in Paris and then in Padua to dissect human bodies without limitations and found many problems with Galen's conclusions. Vesalius believed that Galen had never had the opportunity to dissect humans and therein lies the problem of his anatomical misconceptions (although, as noted earlier, this is up for debate). Vesalius was a product of his time. At the heart of the Renaissance, he was exploring new worlds, opening new doors, as artists and musicians contributed to the rebirth of the arts and took them to previously untouched heights, Vesalius did the same with his anatomical and illustrative book *De Humani Corporis Fabrica* (On the fabric of the human body). The book itself was a thing of beauty. Beneath the handcrafted, elegant spine, the illustrations lived on the page in the flow of curved lines of muscle and hand-drawn smooth edges of bone. In the mid–1500s Vesalius traveled across Europe and learned, wrote, taught, and pushed medical boundaries—the acts of a true Renaissance man. He became obsessed with his book from 1540 to 1542, and when it was published it was immediately recognized as a major and dramatic contribution to the medical community and the medical revelations of the time, as was the release of its revision in 1555—Vesalius continued to dissect and inspect between the release of the first edition and second edition, and the second edition corrected a lot of what he learned to be errors in the first edition.

In chapter 6, "On the Eight Bones of the Head and the Sutures Connecting Them," the aesthetic fruits of commissioning Renaissance artists to draw the images within the book glowed from the page. The shading and bossing and edging not only were beautiful but also jumped off the page as if their edges and curves could fall forward onto the lap of the reader, something unseen to this point in medical diagramming and art. Figures 1 through 3 detail the parietal bones (with the sagittal suture running between them), the skull cut away and shown from the side to reveal the its two layers (the *lamina externa* and *lamina interna* or the inner and outer skull) as well as the spongy barrier between the two (the diploe), and the natural shape of the skull when all things are normal. The drawings are precise. They show, in progression, the bigger shapes, such as the parietal bone, then move to their makeup, and then move to how the skull should look on a developed human being, but it's the fourth diagram or series of diagrams that detailed the anatomical nature of the cranial sutures in such detail that they are noted as exceptional and groundbreaking.

He begins with an illustration of *sutura coronalis* (Latin for "crown" and Greek for "wreath"—both sit on the front of the skull), shown from both the left and right sides of the anterior skull. He then shows the *sutura lambdoidea,* which resembles the Greek capital letter *L* (lambda), which is shaped like an upside-down *V*, also described as the tree suture. Next, he details a squiggly suture from the tip of the lambda-shaped suture (the edge of the upside-down V) to the front of the coronalis suture—the *sutura sagittalis,* thick and long, runs the length of the head in the diagram, squiggling jaggedly from right to left like a mellow heartbeat on an EKG machine, and looks to hold everything together, the whole skull. In the following figures he outlines the *sutura squamosa* that runs thin and wavy above the ears and connects the pterion (the point connected to the sphenoparietal suture) and the temporal squama (the upper part of the temporal bone). With the same detail he illustrates the "interval of adhesion [*sutura parietomastoidea*] … extending from the lambdoid suture to the true squamous adhesion, which shows a construction not of plates lying upon each other, but a genuine suture." He then outlines, as if taken by a camera, the bones of the skull that are connected by the sutures, the left (*os parietale sinister),* right (*os parietale dexter),* front (*os frontale),* back, or occiput, (*os occipitale),* and the left temporal bone.

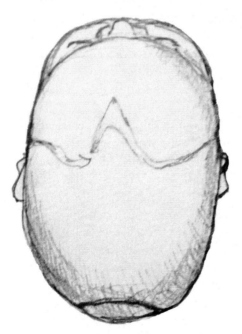

The skull with sagittal synostosis (scaphocephaly) (courtesy of Sean Davis).

Vesalius and his artists go much farther into the detail of the skull and document the smallest of sutures. For example, their pencils shade in all of the miniature sutures that line and connect the sphenoid bone to the larger bones of the skull, and as we have found out in this book, these smaller sutures, while rare, will be fused at birth as well and are just as problematic to the overall growth of the brain as any of the larger sutures, like tiny anchors holding a large boat from moving, and as the tide rises, the boat, hung up by one tiny anchor at one end, will eventually lean into the water. In the fifth group of figures, Vesalius flips the skull over and shows all of the sutures from the inside of the skull in the same detail as from the outside of the skull, like looking into the soul of a corpse.

Vesalius was, and still is, revered for his work and his book that gave the medical world a deeper insight into the body and, for the purpose of this book, the sutures that wind their way through our skulls and connect the bones that cover the human brain. He was the first to recognize the importance of open sutures. He went on to talk about the sutures of naturally shaped heads that have clear openings and an H-shape design created by the sagittal suture and the coronal and lambdoid sutures. Interestingly, he takes time within the book to debunk the myths that men's and women's skulls are "not always" different in structure and nature, a not too uncommon myth that had floated in the study of anatomy up until that point and possibly after.

Vesalius uses a larger part of the chapter 6 to write about sutureless heads, which he terms "unnatural heads," and as I rub my head over my lumps and bumps of scars, the last thing I want to be seen as is unnatural, and I believe every mother who looks down at her child with craniosynostosis feels her child is the most natural and beautiful child in the world, but that is something to discuss in later chapters of this book. Vesalius goes into great detail on the unnatural formation of the skull when the sutures are closed, the first intimate description of the lack of sutures in medical history, and he, laying the skull down in different angles, describes how the skull becomes deformed when the sagittal, lambdoid, coronal, and metopic sutures are closed. The descriptions are interesting, but this is where Vesalius got it wrong. The shapes that he describes are illustrated incorrectly, the skull taking shape in ways that do not depict proper expansion of the skull near the closed suture.

Another three hundred years would pass before knowledge of suture ossification would advance. As the son of a medical professor, Adolph Wilhelm Otto grew up in Germany's medical community in the late 1700s and early 1800s, nearly three hundred years after Vesalius illustrated, in great detail, the presence of the sutures and the impact of closed sutures on the skull and brain. Otto, a bright young anatomist and doctor who flourished, like his father, in the Frankfurt halls of medicine, was elected to multiple prestigious boards, panels, and presidencies throughout his tenure in the medical community. Known for his dedication to scientific and medical exploration and also known for his concentration on his favorite studies and routes of medical exploration, Otto never neglected his favorite study of teratology—the study, rooted in biology, of diagnosing, recognizing the causes of, and looking for solutions to congenital malformations, those that are present at birth. He looked at these malformations in plants, animals, and, in his term, "human monsters." His descriptive work of what he found is revered, but according to many, he failed to look at his subjects in a heavily physiological way or under the microscope. What he did do, however, was provide even more insight into the sutures of the skull, their importance, and how the early ossification of them, craniosynostosis, can affect brain development, taking it one step further than Vesalius by not just describing a skull with closed sutures but also recognizing that when they close is just as important as their being closed. In his book *A Compendium of Human & Comparative Pathological Anatomy*, Otto focuses, like his predecessors, on the makeup on the human body from head to toe, describing the nervous and skeletal systems in great detail, but his contributions come in recognition and heavy descriptions of the congenital malformations. He notes with immediacy in his section "Of the Bones of the Head" that the human skull is very deficient because of the multitude of bones that make up the skull and need to work together to create a normal skull. At birth, Otto notes, the amount of bones increases based on the number of sutural bones present. He discusses the lambdoid, coronal, and squamus suture briefly and notes that they are rarely symmetrical and that there can be hundreds of bones associated with these sutural bones. What he means by this is not entirely clear, but he quickly moves past these sutural bones and focuses on the fontanel bone, or the lack of the fontanel suture. If the coronal sutures are in place, Otto was describing the closure of the metopic suture that created one solid bone in the front of the skull and therefore recognizing and defining craniosynostosis as we know it today—the premature closure of one or more sutures.

Otto, much to my anger but giving him the benefit of his time and place in the world and the belief that he studied deformations with good intentions, called those born without the properly opened sutures "monsters." His monsters, he believed, were created by the premature closure of the sutures, as he notes in this section, and the closure explained dropsy of the brain or watery head, rickets (a disease of children characterized by a large head, crooked spine and limbs, tumid abdomen, and general debility, often accompanied with precocious mental faculties), and cretinism (an endemic disease common in Switzerland and other mountainous countries, characterized by goiter, stinted growth, swelled abdomen, wrinkled skin, wan complexion, vacant and stupid countenance, misshapen cranium, idiocy, and comparative insensibility). The definitions of cretinism and dropsy of the brain at least temper today's connotations of those words. All of this, according to Otto, comes about from the misshapenness of the head—this seems to be an early indication of the devastation of internal cranial pressure on the brain that can lead to numerous problems that stretch through the mental, physical, and physiological development of children. He describes the skull as unusually flat, angular, long, broad, or too round, all legitimate descriptions of the consequences of craniosynostosis. Otto's descriptions were highly insightful and lead to many of the things families in this book have faced, including thinning or thickening of the skull, even absence of necessary skull bone, because of the fused suture and its pulling toward one point, even noting that at times the bone can become so thin that it looks transparent. He tied this thinness to dropsy of the head, rickets, and cretinism, and these many be symptoms of the thinning out of the skull in places because the bone has ossified in other parts, but more important, he mentions that the bone in these thin areas may never ossify at all, as you will see in some of the children in later chapters of this book.

Where Otto begins to fascinate, having written about craniosynostosis nearly two hundred years ago and having very little to go on except for the writings of Vesalius and Galen, with no large medical team of researchers, lies within his larger assessments of the birth defect and the thickening of the skull above the closed suture. The hypertrophy (the outward increase in volume or size) of the skull, commonly associated with craniosynostosis, according to Otto, is far worse a symptom than that of the thinning of the skull, mainly because he felt it led to the hypertrophy of the brain as well. His analysis of "why" craniosynostosis occurs, honestly, is not that far behind our current-day hypotheses. He notes that sometimes it happens because of placement in the womb and sometimes it just happens—this is just about where we are today. We know that placement may cause some early sutures' closures, and we know that some are closed by a certain gene (According to a 2013 study by the Seattle Children's Research Institute, together with an international team of scientists and clinicians from twenty-two other institutions, a genome-wide association study identifies susceptibility loci for nonsyndromic sagittal craniosynostosis near BMP2 and within BBS9), but we really don't know "why" that gene develops in some and not others. From there, Otto, and this must be taken with skepticism, relates insanity or the insane to having thick skulls in certain areas. Putting that aside, he recognizes that makeup of the bone in these thick areas is typically very healthy and stable, very solid, unlike the makeup of the bone in the thin, transparent areas, and he discusses the connection between the bones of the "insane" to be irregularly thick and dense, talking about the sutures that hold the thick parts of the skull together. He mentions, briefly, the problem of some of the sutures never closing but quickly dismisses it as rare before moving on to the more common and problematic issue with the sutures: anchylosis (abnormal adhesion and rigidity of the bones of a joint). Otto, without years and years of medical research and observation performed by a team, says that this anchylosis occurs most commonly in the sagittal suture but clarifies by stating that although it is most common in the sagittal suture, it is not a rarity in other sutures. Our current knowledge backs this up with long-term studies and gathering of numbers nationally and internationally. If that weren't impressive enough, the nineteenth-century doctor notes that, at times, all sutures can be closed congenitally, pansynostosis. Through my travels and research, however, I have yet to find an insane person who developed his/her insanity through the ossification of his/her sutures, but Otto's observations could only be deemed remarkable, especially since he was criticized by his peers for not picking up a microscope.

During the 1800s, around the same time Otto was observing and writing, Josef Hyrtl, owner of one of the largest skull collections in the world at the time, recognized, in more depth than Otto, the early closure of the sutures lead to deformity of the skull. Hyrtl's collection of skulls was believed to be populated, mostly, by the collection of skulls from paupers and grave robbers in the mid–1800s. He donated his skulls to the Mütter Museum in Pennsylvania, where most of those skulls can still be found today. Many of the skulls are labeled "Cretin," as described earlier, and their descriptions are noted as "Cretin [Swiss in origin with a misshapen head]; premature closure of the coronal suture" or "Porter [occupation]; demonstrates scaphocephaly (keeled or boat-shaped head) [premature closure of the sagittal suture]" or "Robber [occupation]. Court martialed. Depressed nasal root; persistent frontal suture." Hyrtl's collection can still be visited in Pennsylvania at the Mütter Museum, and he is credited with advancing the study of cranial deformations caused by craniosynostosis by amassing such a large collection of skulls and preserving them for others to view and study.

It was Rudolph Virchow who first classified the different types of craniosynotosis and the terminology of their deformations that we still use today. Virchow confirmed that theory that the side of the head of the affected suture is affected by the suture and therefore its growth is restricted, and as happens in medical science, some of his findings have been disputed, but for the most part, his work served as one of the most significant backbones for what would come next in the evolution of the knowledge of sutures, closed sutures, and craniosynostosis: surgery. Virchow first defined scapholocephalic (boat-shaped) skulls, describing the closure of the most common suture, the sagittal suture. Along with the description of the effects of the premature closure of the sagittal suture, he also, within his descriptions, coined the terms "trigonocephaly" for the shape of the head created by a closed metopic suture, as the forehead would grow triangularly outward above the brow line, "anterior pla-giocephaly" for the growth of the unilateral coronal synostosis, as the head would flatten and shift downward, "brachyocephaly" for bilateral coronal syn-ostosis (both coronal sutures fully or partially fused, which creates a shortening and widening of the skull as well as a heightening of the skull, and the closing of the lambdoid suture, which could be bilateral or unilateral, the bilateral closing (both sides of the lambdoid closing) typically found in patients with a much more serious syndrome. Virchow's law more precisely defines the effects of a closed suture: when premature suture closure occurs, growth of the skull is typically restricted perpendicular to the fused suture and enhanced in a plane parallel to it, thus trying to provide space for the fast-growing brain. In other words, the side of the skull that is connected to the suture grows either forward, backward, or sideways at a ninety-degree angle straight out from the suture. The skull parallel, or alongside, the suture must compensate and there-fore grows outward by growing in a manner least resistant to the growing skull.

His proclamation that the skull grows along a parallel plane to that of the fused suture was revolutionary and correct—some very recent develop-ments in research blame the dura matter associated with the closed suture for the early closure, but this body of evidence is still in the testing and hypothesis stage. Virchow's contribution to medical science, however, extends much fur-ther into the annals of medical history and its progression. Virchow, the son of a farmer from Germany, loved the natural sciences, and from his childhood he had a very strong inclination toward botany and biology and their relation-ship. He was an army physician who would go on to found, along with his col-league Benino Reinhardt, *Virchow's Archives of Anatomy and Pathology.* The journal still lives as one of the leading medical journals today, and at its birth Virchow changed the way the medical community viewed illness and disease. Virchow taught his students to "think microscopically," four of his students going on to found Johns Hopkins Hospital. He is most well known for rec-ognizing that, for the most part, when an organism gets sick only some cells within the organism get sick, launching the vast, ever-expanding, and myste-rious field of pathology. This revelation changed medicine. It made it possible for physicians to attribute certain anatomical changes to very specific diag-noses, making treatment much more effective. He was the first to recognize that all diseases come from the change in normal cells. This introduction of pathology into the medical community changed the way we view disease today and, as linked to craniosynostosis, still leads us to our biggest question that is still not answered, pathologically at least: what cells or change in cells cause craniosynostosis.

Another half century later, the observations of Hippocrates, the dissection of Galen, the artistic contributions of Vesalius, the recognition of no sutures from Otto, and the law of Virchow would lead Dr. Odilon Marc Lannelongue, a French surgeon, to take the first steps toward the correction of craniosynostosis by sawing into the head of a man with a fused sagittal suture, notching the adjacent areas of the skull, and pulling out about two inches of skull from the anterior fontanel to the posterior fontanel. Lannelongue performed, according to most, the first strip craniectomy by pulling the bone bilaterally along the sagittal suture in 1890. Surgical intervention, previous to Lannelongue, was not considered necessary until the birth defect was linked directly to blindness and other neurological problems that were evident through simple observation of shared symptoms. Lannelongue's method focused on the release of the suture by simply taking a bilateral strip for sagittal synostosis, and he believed release of the suture would give better results than resection of the bone (removing the bone completely in the affected area).

Two years later, in San Francisco, Dr. Lane operated on a young boy. Lane removed the stenosed sagittal suture along with a lateral strip of the parietal bone—the large bones that line the sagittal suture—bilaterally, but the child died fourteen hours after the surgery due to complications with anesthesia. But it could have been infection, blood loss, or a number of other complications that came with early cranial surgery. Lane's decision to operate on the child was not a rash one. Lane told the story of a scared and desperate mother who approached him through the post and begged him to open up her child's head, saying, "Can you not unlock my poor child's brain and let it grow?" This sentiment, this pleading, this recognition by a parent that her child needed help, echoes today in the waiting rooms of all the parents of children born with craniosynostosis. It took four years for Lane to decide to perform the surgery. Once the surgery was performed, Lane took the boy into the operating room and released the suture by performing the second strip craniectomy to correct craniosynostosis to that day. The boy lost his life, and the mother lost her boy.

In a very brief article published in the *Journal of the American Medical Association,* Lane wrote about the women, his diagnosis of the boy, and his procedures: "Early in the month of August, 1888, I received a letter from a lady residing in the interior of California, stating that she desired to consult me concerning her infant, then nearly 9 months of age, which presented signs of mental imbecility. At the time appointed for the consultation, the lady presented herself with her infant. The child, otherwise in good health and well nourished, was decidedly microcephalic. The cranium was symmetrical, and only deviated from normal type in the smallness of its volume. The mother stated that at birth the anterior fontanelle was wholly closed, and the posterior one nearly so."

To say that the procedure was experimental for its time would be an understatement, but Lane, listening to a mother who never, it can be assumed, never had access to Virchow, Hippocrates, or Vesalius, looked at her son and his inability to keep up with other children, even at 9 months old, and begged for a physician to help her out, proceeded with the surgery. The mother, with no medical training or background in anatomy, knew not only that there was something wrong with her child but also where the problem was—in his sutures—and she became her child's advocate, and for the first time in the medical history of craniosynostosis a mother (a parent) did whatever she could, did not take "no" for an answer, and handed her child over to a surgeon with the hopes of giving the boy a better life. It seems that mothers have always been the same, and this mother, it must be noted, alongside all of the researchers and physicians who contributed to the medical growth and push of medical knowledge over the centuries, became the first necessary link in the medical history chain of cranisynostosis: she became the first mother who worried about the repair while her son was taken away, and she was the first believer that her child could have a better life if only his head could be unlocked so his brain could grow. Sadly, she would be the first to lose a child that day, fourteen hours after she let him go.

Although these attempts were failures, the strip craniectomy became very popular within the community of surgeons and spread wildly across the cranium landscape. Surgical texts illustrating and describing various techniques for craniectomies popped up all over the world, but the medical world got ahead of itself. First, researchers believe that most of the patients suffered from microcephaly, like the young boy operated on in San Francisco, instead of craniosynostosis—physicians probably diagnosed them as the same congenital birth defect at the time. The second major setback arose from the recognition of the birth defect and the timing of the procedure. In other words, the synostosis was not recognized in infants or wasn't seen as a medical problem, and as the children grew they developed neurological developmental delays and deficits, so when the child (or adult) developed major neurological and very noticeable problems the synostosis had already taken hold of the skull and the brain and once operated on the suture re-fused relatively quickly after the reconstruction—the fix was only temporary. With all of these complications, the surgical practice of releasing supposed cases of craniosynostosis would run into its worst opponent, which was necessary and as common then as it is today: peer review—in this case, very harsh peer review.

Dr. Abraham Jacobi, a physician whom many historians call the founder of pediatrics, was the first to spearhead specialization in diagnosing and treating children and infants differently than adults. Jacobi himself was considered a rebel in his times and reshaped the landscape of children through his lifelong work by venturing into new medical territory previously undiscovered, so he was not against forging ahead and trying new things to make the world a better place for his patients. Born in Germany in 1830 and moving to the United States in 1853 to avoid persecution for progressive political activism in a very conservative German society, he published hundreds of pieces in the major New York medical journals, and it was these publications that focused on pediatric care that spawned the specialty in pediatrics. He was the first full hire at the New York Medical College to teach pediatric pathology, as well as the first in the United States, and he began to change not only what was taught but also how it was taught by flipping medical instruction on its ear; he founded the pediatric clinic next. Jacobi spent the rest of his life pushing the pediatric specialty knob further and further until he eventually founded the medical pediatric section of the American Medical Association and the pediatric section of the New York Academy of Medicine, in 1880 and 1885 respectively.

So when Dr. Jacobi, arguably the most renowned pediatrician in the world, with no doubt in the United States, stood up in front of the who's who of the medical community at the American Academy of Pediatrics, having studied the thirty-three surgical outcomes for strip craniectomies and finding that fifteen out of the thirty-three patients died, and denounced the practice of releasing fused sutures, people listened. His speech did not pull punches:

> The relative impunity of operative interference accomplished by modern asepsis and antisepsis has developed an undue tendency to, and rashness in, handling the knife. The hands take too frequently the place of brains.... Is it sufficient glory to don a white apron and swing a carbonized knife, and is therein a sufficient indication to let daylight into a deformed cranium and on top of the hopelessly defective brain, and to proclaim a success because the victim consented not to die of the assault? Such rash feats of indiscriminate surgery ... are stains on your hands and sins on your soul. No ocean of soap and water will clean those hands, no power of corrosive sublimate will disinfect the souls.

He drilled into the practices of those surgeons like Lane and Lannelongue for being hasty in their decision to open up the heads of children for the simple reason that they could. He derided them for making the prognosis for those with closed sutures worse, taking it from "defective" to death. When he thrashed at their very souls and illustrated the blood on their hands in a speech that was presumably delivered with the fervor of a preacher warning his flock about the mouths of hell, the pediatric community virtually stopped performing craniectomies for the next three to four decades—and, for the most part, they probably should have if for the simple reason that doctors hadn't been able to distinguish between microcephaly and craniosynostosis.

Doctors in the 1930s and 1940s had a lot of success with new methods of craniectomies. They recognized that the simplest procedure worked just as well as or better than more complicated procedures to release the synosed suture; they found that if children were opened up before two months old they suffered less damage to the skull, had a higher mortality rate, and had a better cosmesis outcome (they looked better as they grew). The doctors found that the earlier the surgery the better the surgery, as the pliability of the skull heightens the success of the surgery. But their work was not free of complications. While their immediate surgical outcomes were successful, their long-term results were not. When their patients got older, the affected suture reossified and this resossification led to large, complicated surgeries, similar to complicated surgeries that are commonplace and safe today, to fix the bridging of the stubborn skull over the artificial suture that had been opened. The skull took back its territory quickly and without hesitation, growing and growing until it did what it had always intended to do: close.

Just like Dr. Jacobi did, another prestigious doctor of the time weighed in on surgery to correct craniosynostosis. Dr. Harvey Cushing in the early twentieth century, when doctors were having some success with early-age craniectomies, asked, like Dr. Jacobi, if the opening of the skull to release the suture was a responsible and ethical thing to do—just because surgeons could do it. To those in the medical community, Dr. Cushing is the founder of the specialty of neurosurgery (very similar to Dr. Jacobi), and like Jacobi, he doubted the virtue in surgical intervention, at first. The morbidity rate of children who were operated on in the first third of the twentieth century was still very high, so Cushing shied away from doing the surgery himself and did not agree with the idea to operate on children. During the beginning of Cushing's practice, secondary microcephaly was still being misdiagnosed as craniosynostosis. Cushing believed, like Jacobi, that linear craniectomies were sad cases of "juror operandi running away with surgical judgment." He also felt that unless the patient had epilepsy or hydrocephephalus there would be no benefit to a craniectomy—moreover, he thought it would be negligent and hurtful, especially considering the nearly 50 percent morbidity rate. He stated very clearly in his speech about surgery of the head, "There has been a high mortality in these operations, and though death cannot be lamented, the surgeon is not a barbarian to execute the helpless." At the time, blood loss was credited with the loss of most children in the OR, as transfusions were rudimentary, unsterile, and unsafe, so when a child came into the OR with limited blood it only took the smallest loss of blood to put the child at risk of death.

As noted, it was in the 1920s when the doctors revisited craniectomies, this time just removing the synosed suture with success. Cushing, recognizing later in his career in the mid–1920s that there could be some developmental issues connected with craniosynostosis, tried his hand at a handful of surgeries and recorded some successes as well as some less successful craniectomies, but with Cushing and other prominent surgeons like him as very admired mouthpieces, it opened the door again to more surgeries and more exploration into surgical procedures, and with this open door and continued effort progress was bound to walk in.

In the 1930s surgeons began, as a large community, to see surgery as a promising endeavor for those born with cranioysnostosis. To say that the surgery had become routine at the time would be an overstatement, but surgeons began to operate more and more often, and the mortality rate began to drop quickly and steadily over the next few decades. In the late 1940s Dr. Alexander Ingraham and his crew of researchers studied fifty patients with craniosynostosis—forty-four of them had craniectomies to treat their synosed suture. They found then that if all the proper measures were taken—proper anesthesia, proper management of blood loss—then the mortality rate of these patients was quite small. This was good news. It ushered in a new era of craniofacial management through surgical techniques. Five years later, in 1954, Ingraham and fellow surgeon and teacher D.D. Matson found that patients' aesthetics improved along with the surgery as well, so, in their medical textbook they listed aesthetic benefits as another supporting reason for craniectomies to remove the synosed suture in children. At that point in medical time, the craniofacial world changed.

For the first time in the correction of the synosed suture, the word "cosmetic" came into play, and, even though this word has caused more heartbreak and controversy over the years—parents hear the word and doubt not only their doctor's intentions but, more important, their own intentions in subjecting their child to reconstructive surgery—in the 1950s, 1960s, and 1970s, the term "cosmetic" and cosmetic indications for craniosynostosis were termed and used correctly because the safety of the procedure had to be ensured before any discussion of aesthetic improvement happened. Cosmetics was a bonus, not a prognosis, and this is how families should still see the use of the word "cosmetic" today, as a bonus of the corrective and reconstructive surgery.

At Children's Hospital of Boston (CHB), Drs. Matson and Ingraham tried tackling other challenges. While the strip craniectomy for very young infants had become more and more successful over the first few decades since reintroduction to the surgical world, older children who underwent surgery weren't having the same positive and consistent results for two main reasons: death and reossification of the released suture. Drs. Matson and Ingraham lined the edges of the stripped bone with polyethylene following the craniectomy. Two other surgeons, Drs. Simmons and Peyton, placed tantalum foil between the edges of the bone like a buffer to keep the bone from coming together. Both of these methods did not survive long in the surgical world. Both led to infection and reossification. Drs. Anderson and Johnson used Zenker's solution in 1956, which helped cauterize the incision, the bone, and any other elements opened up, but, sadly, the placement of the solution on the brain caused seizures in children. With the advances in blood transfusion and anesthesia, surgical developments become much easier to come by. Matson and Ingraham extended the strip craniectomy by cutting out the pericranium and excising bone from the healthy sutures as well. The removal of the pericranium helped eliminate the reossification and the extra bone excised from the healthy sutures helped with the overall growth of the fused suture.

A thirty-six-year review of the procedure, beginning in 1930 and ending in 1966, revealed that the mortality rate of the procedure was at much less than 1 percent at 0.39 percent, the morbidity rate (patients who were deemed unhealthy within the operative population after surgery) was 14 percent, and those with undesirable sequelae (having shown an undesirable aftereffect from surgery) hung around half of a percent at 0.58 percent. Over that thirty-year span, while nearly one out of six still struggled with their health after the surgery, fewer than 1 percent lost their lives or acquired problems due to having surgery, coming in at just two deaths in 519 surgeries performed. While this is a low number for the group, for the parents of those who lost their children it must be emphasized that their number is a 100 percent mortality rate, and this cannot be overemphasized. For the most part, however, these numbers come from the opening of the most commonly closed suture, the sagittal suture, as it was the easiest to release through the strip craniectomy and Matson and Ingraham's craniosynostectomy became very widespread for the release of the synosed suture, but these techniques had limitations for sutures outside the most commonly closed sagittal suture.

During the span of time from the early 1900s to the late 1960s, while strip craniectomies were becoming safer and safer and more and more common, many other advancements happened in the study and practice of craniofacial surgery. With war comes progress. During the First and Second World

Wars, advancements in craniofacial surgery pushed forward in unison with the soldiers on the battlefield, grappling forward over lines that were previously impermeable. Soldiers were carried into the medical tents and hospitals who had been subjected to massive facial and skull injuries. These trauma-related injuries, under the guise of battle, laid the groundwork for a growth in craniofacial surgery that treated facial and skull bone injuries and led to reconstructive practices in soldiers. These practices, scraped up off the remnants of war-torn medical sheets, were adopted by surgeons who dealt with the correction of congenital birth defects and deformations of the cranium and face.

After the war, Dr. Paul Tessier in France began developing new, advanced techniques in the craniofacial world that would not only relate directly to releasing the sutures to give the brain its natural path and to give the child the best possible chance to avoid any developmental delays or permanent restrictions but also help to shape the head to give the child the best possible chance of looking good. His predecessors learned that the bones of the face and skull could be reshaped, pulled from the wreckage of trauma, to re-create a cranium close to what was there before the trauma had occurred. Tessier had a hands-on view of what happened in medical hospitals, having spent his last year of medical services in a German prison camp as a military prisoner of war. His studies were not in plastic or reconstructive surgery but rather in general surgery, orthopedics, and ophthalmology, but all of these studies lent themselves nearly perfectly to what he saw and gained a passion for during his time at the Center for Maxillofacial Surgery of the Military Region of Paris Hospital in Puteaux. A year after his time at the Military Region of Paris Hospital in Puteaux, the center was moved to another hospital in Paris, where he became intrigued with the practice of plastic surgery and burn care.

Dr. Tessier, having seen firsthand the use of bone to help reshape traumatized victims, saw that his predecessors and their patients suffered relapses in their treatment, meaning that the reshaping of their faces and skulls did not stay as the doctors wished they would. Tessier, as his obituary in the *Indian Journal of Plastic Surgery* states, reshaped the way plastic surgery would be seen from his time on and "the fact that Cranio-facial Surgery is so popular the world over is an ample testimony to the greatness of this colossal man of surgical sciences," and here's why.

Tessier saw the advances and downfalls of his predecessors and decided to do something different. First, he introduced the practice of intentionally fractured osteotomies. He saw that by purposefully breaking the bones of the face and cranium surgeons would have more material to work with in the reshaping of the skulls and faces of those born with congenital malformations—instead of using the pieces of the puzzle given to him, he figured out that he would have a lot better chance of creating a masterpiece if he created the puzzle pieces himself. Second, to that leap forward in plastic surgery vision, he saw that the reason his mentors had high failure rates was because the bone reshaped was unstable, so Tessier introduced bone grafting to stabilize the bones by placing the grafts in the skull to steady the gaps during and after the surgery.

In 1967, just nine short years before my birth and strip craniectomy, he stood in front of room full of peers from across the globe and performed these techniques. Then, he asked for them to vote. He asked them to vote on the future of his practices and if these new practices belonged in the practice of surgery. The response was not just positive; it was so positive that craniofacial surgery became a new specialty in the profession. From that point, Dr. Tessier packed his bags in the early 1970s and traveled to Boston, to Chicago, to Houston, and to New York City to demonstrate what his techniques brought to the world of plastic surgery and craniofacial surgery. It would not take long before plastic surgeons and craniofacial surgeons would stand next to neurosurgeons in the operating room and work on children with craniosynostosis, a place where neurosurgeons had stood alone for nearly a century.

Just a few years later, I would be born. From that time in the early 1970s to the present, advances in suture release would blossom like the wildflowers that flowed through the mountains that looked down on my home in Utah in 1976.

It seems like surgical advances—more accurately, a breadth of surgical techniques were pioneered—in craniosynostosis diagnosis and repair were born in near correlation with my birth. First, doctors were starting to diagnose children earlier, and this early diagnosis gave options of different types of surgical procedures that were highly beneficial for the next generation of children born with one or multiple fused sutures.

Drs. David Staffenberg from the NYU Medical Center and Jeffrey Fearon of the Craniofacial Center in Dallas, two of the most well-respected craniofacial surgeons in the country, look at these last thirty to forty years from the craniofacial perspective and give their perspective on where we are now and how far we've come, both breaking the surgical history and current state of medical advancements into laymen's terms, or how they would for their patients—treating the people who sit in front of them as intelligent listeners as well as shocked and scared parents.

Looking back at his predecessors, Dr. Staffenberg said:

> There are plenty of options for how this is treated, and we see these babies, the variables that are important include the age of the baby at the time of their evaluation and the severity of the physical findings. In other words,

how bad is their head shape changed? And fortunately, because I think there's more awareness, we can definitely see over the years that babies are getting to us at a younger age, which then is a great thing because it presents options for us. It allows us to consider other kinds of surgery. I had a baby who came from Ohio because [his] parents were very on the ball, [his] parents did quick research and the operation was done. There's a history of over a hundred years, called a craniectomy. And you know what I'm talking about, just basically going in and removing the suture, the area of the seized bones for the long rectangle shape. Well, leaving that part of the brain exposed, no bone over it, skin is closed, end of the operation, and what we know of that operation, done that way, is that it was successful in about 15 percent of patients. And so that technique was abandoned.

Dr. Fearon looks at the years and the current state of medical advancements from a different but similar perspective:

Neurosurgeons saw a fused suture and thought the way to treat it would be to cut it out, to release it, but I should back up a little bit. The skull grows in two ways basically; it grows by dissolving bone in the inside and laying new bone on the outside so like layers of bark on a tree it gets bigger, but that form of growth is probably too slow early on in life when the brain is just growing "gangbusters" and so you also have sutural growth so the skull grows, but there are different bones where they come together, the joints are called sutures, and as the brain gets bigger it pulls those joints apart and that stretch tells the skull that you got to get bigger. And so if you look under the microscope next to a suture, all the dividing bones are really close to the suture and as we now know today about 1 in 1,700 kids are born with one of these sutures fused shot, but it's likely that at least three things can cause sutural fusions. One is certain gene mutations, but they're less common forms of craniosynostosis, and others are certain drugs and they're even more rare. Like, for instance, valproic acid, also Depakote, in this country is a drug that's given to mothers for seizures and can cause early closure of the metopic suture and trigonocephaly and a lot of excess anti-acid use. Some pediatricians would tell their moms to give their babies a lot of anti-acids and that can fuse them.

So there are a bunch of metabolic things that can do it [too], but the science today suggests the most common reason for it is the infant gets its head caught in a tight position—I should say the fetus in the womb—and that prevents the skull from expanding and that may be the reason that most kids get craniosynostosis. And there are a bunch of animal models to suggest this is the case. If you prolong a rat pregnancy for a day or two, 80 percent of rats or more will be born with some sutures fusion. It's more common that craniosynostosis happens with twins than singletons. We know it's more common in boys than girls and some research suggests the male hormone testosterone makes sutures a little stickier.

But the suture is a pretty complicated region anatomically, the brain lives inside this water balloon called the dura and it floats in this dura, and we know that chemical messengers are going back and forth all the time. When the suture becomes fused it becomes disconnected from the dura and so those messengers aren't going back and forth and when a surgeon goes in and takes a strip of bone out they're not creating a functioning suture again.

Now if you take enough strips of bone out in enough ways the bones can float around and maybe allow the dura to expand, but if you just, say, with sagittal synostosis cut the sagittal suture out the bone on the side only is going to allow it to expand a little bit and it depends upon the age how much it allows it to expand and then it's not going to get much bigger, so it's only a partial release. And then, as I told you, if the dura is young, if the kids are young, the dura which covers the brain is really where the new bones comes from, it can put bony bridges across in two weeks and then after that two weeks you're re-fused you've got little bridges across and the whole thing can re-fuse with bone or maybe just parts will. And as the kids get older and older you're going to get fewer bony bridges.

With families today, however, the Internet provides a slough of information on what types of surgeries should be performed, what are the best surgeries, and how the doctors should proceed. This excess of available information is very positive when it comes to diagnosis, but it can be make things difficult when it comes to treatment, as parents believe they have found the best technique online for their child but fail to understand that every child is different and, therefore, every surgical decision is different, and, most of the time, parents feel that the smallest surgery is the best surgery when this is not the case—the best surgery for their child is the best surgery for their child, size notwithstanding.

Dr. Staffenberg notes:

So for, for craniosynostosis and the different kinds of surgery that are involved, you know, I think that in a sense, all of the surgeons will talk about the difference between the neurosurgical involvement and the plastic surgery involvement. The plastic surgeon is typically referred to as the craniofacial surgeon, but all of the surgeons basically have, at their disposal, essentially the same ingredients as another surgeon, but their recipes may be different—how they use the ingredients may be a little different, and for sure, just like going to a restaurant, you know you may go to one restaurant and find their recipe is better than another, but personal taste may be a little different. But, now, I think that's probably not, a bad analogy for that, because we're all taught the same skills. The magic is really how we sort of combine them and I find it to be very, very easy to design a very complex, difficult operation for a problem and much harder to design a small, safe, and yet effective solution so, you know, the tendency, I think, for a lot of physicians—at least again, this is sort of from my perspective over the years—it seems like there's a gravitational pull for surgeons to do the most complex thing and yet that is not necessarily the best solution. The best solution is always the safest and simplest operation that has the greatest chance of giving the results that the patient, the family, and the doctor want. So what does that mean? I have found that there have been patients who have had operations described to them and, you know, everything I'm sort of describing is feedback that I get from patients' families that I see. And they'll say, "Well, there are big operations that we can do, but we're going to do a smaller operation. And we're going to do it because it makes sense that a smaller operation would be safer," and so there's a lot of commonsense thinking involved and so a baby would then go through a simpler, smaller operation.

And then at the end of the operation, even though it's safe, baby's gone through a general anesthetic, baby stays in the hospital, and at the end of the day, when everything's healed, they look the same, or the result is bumpy, or areas of bone have not healed so they're soft bone there. So then where are we? We've now put the baby through surgery and they're no better off than they were before, so that, yes, a simple and safe is really important, but if we're going to do something it has to be something that I feel is going to be successful. I don't want to leave things to chance. This is why endoscopic surgery is not necessarily the best solution for everyone. These are the kinds of things that we talk about all the time, and every time I see a baby who has an issue like this.

I just had a conversation two days ago in the office, a baby from Louisiana with all of the techniques that we have available to us, and parents know that I do this technique and that technique and if I choose one technique, why, why is it that I'm doing it that way? [It would be] easy for me to say, "Because I'm the doctor," but the parents leave at the end of the day and they just feel, fret, "Well, why, why wouldn't he do the other thing?" Nothing makes the parent more uncomfortable than if they don't understand. They'll never be 100 percent. If you're saying that the baby needs an operation and the baby doesn't need an operation, they're never going to be 100 percent comfortable; they're always going to be nervous, but you want them to be as comfortable as possible, so that open, sort of, dialogue and encouraging them to ask questions is very, very important.

What cannot be disregarded or underplayed is how far we've come, how safe the surgery has become, and how craniosynostosis is a major birth defect of the skull but a major birth defect that can be fixed and, most of the time, fixed successfully. This is where the hope in the following chapters, stories of families from across the country, lives, but Dr. Staffenberg put it better than I ever could:

> One of the things that I really enjoy about this [craniosynostosis] is that it, in the majority of cases, is a problem that can be fixed. I mean, as a young parent, you almost can't imagine facing a more complicated or abstract problem, and not to minimize babies and patients who have heart problems, cancer, or tumors, but there are lots and lots of horrendous things that we wouldn't even want to imagine as young parents, but the fact that we can take this [craniosynostosis] and we can sit down with parents and give them some sort of a mini-fellowship so that they understand the birth defect and medical procedure enough to know what's happening with their baby, and they can also understand why it is we do what we do to make it better, is what I really love

about my work. After all, in the vast majority of cases, we can simply make it sort of vanish. We can make it something that stays in the rearview mirror for these parents and children. No matter what technique we use for surgery, there's going to be a scar somewhere. Even if it's never noticed, there is a scar that's permanent, but other than that, the problem goes away. Every once in a while a parent will ask and I'm not quite sure how to answer the question, "Does the baby *have* craniosynostosis?" The great part is that it's not something that requires medication and, for the most part, they can say "the baby *had* craniosynostosis at birth." It's not like diabetes. When the patient is treated well [properly], even if you're successful, they still have diabetes. You know, the insulin can *control* it, diet can *control* it, but with craniosynostosis when it's treated successfully it becomes something you had and it is no longer there and, in the majority of cases, we're, thankfully, talking about what doctors call simple craniosynostosis for single suture craniosynostosis and, thankfully, only a minority of cases are more severe.

Dr. Staffenberg leaned back in his chair and pointed to photo of a young boy who had syndromic craniosyostosis. His eyes and ears were shifted up and down. Even though he had multiple surgeries, his syndromic synostosis was apparent in the photo. Staffenberg stared at the boy's photo for a few seconds longer, and a smile came over his face, a smile of two points of pride: the first seemed to be one of pride in his own work, how he had helped the boy, and the second a pride in the knowledge that, as he knew the boy personally, the boy was doing well. Of course, the depiction of the doctor's smile is speculative, but having spent the morning with him, I bet I' m pretty close. This man cares about his former and current patients. The boy has a very complex case of craniosynostosis, one of those that we would say are genetic, but these are, again, luckily, the rare forms of the birth defect. The majority are in that rearview mirror.

The Fever—
Inside Anesthesia

In 1892, as noted earlier, according to the medical records from the time, after Dr. Lane pulled the stenosed sagittal suture from the child in San Francisco the boy died from complications with anesthesia less than twenty-four hours post-op.

Things have changed. Today, anesthesia is safe. And complications from anesthesia are rare, and anesthesiologists do their best to avoid those complications, especially when they deal with young children like those born with craniosynostosis.

It would be shortsighted to say there are no risks with anesthesia when a surgeon opens up a child's head and either removes bone or reconstructs bone. The child must be put under anesthesia before and during the surgery so the neurosurgeon and plastic surgeon can do their work. According to Dr. Nicole Jeffreys, a pediatric anesthesiologist at Primary Children's Hospital in Salt Lake City, the best anesthesiologists are the ones the surgeons never even know are there because they do their jobs so well, but doing their jobs so well, according to Dr. Jeffreys, must come in the form of obsession because they are dealing with small children.

"You're [as a pediatric anesthesiologist] obsessed with precision," she notes, "You have to be absolutely precise. Everyone in the operating room has to be very vigilant with children."

From a pediatric anesthesiologist's point of view, from the point of a view of a specialist in the pediatric field, families have to know that the anesthesiologist is watching every beat of their child's heart while under anesthesia, watching their child's hematocrit, red blood cell count, and hemoglobin levels, and watching for anything out of the ordinary that sometimes happens with

58

young children, as children's bodies react differently than those of adults under anesthesia.

"Beat by beat by beat, we watch," Dr. Jeffreys says. When there is a problem, anesthesiologists are usually the ones who take care of it, because while the surgeon works, carving into bone, the anesthesiologists focuses on the child's overall well-being.

Surgeons make the decision, along with the families, to perform, typically, one of two types of surgeries: an endoscopic surgery early on in the child's life (usually between two and three months of age) and a larger reconstructive surgery later on in the child's life (usually between nine and eleven months). Once that decision is made, the anesthesiologist must reconcile the risks of both options, and as Dr. Jeffreys describes them, the risks are like comparing apples and oranges—they cannot really be compared because they are different in their procedural nature, from the anesthesiologist's point of view.

When children undergo endoscopic surgery, usually a strip craniectomy, they are typically between the ages of two and three months. At this age they are just exiting their physiologic nadir, so infants are at risk of anemia during their surgery and they have a lower hemoglobin count, so they have much less blood to lose before they enter into risky territory with the necessity of a transfusion, but since the surgeons cut very little bone, the child bleeds much less, so the need for transfusion is very rare, especially in children's hospitals like Primary Children's in Salt Lake City.

The risks for the larger, more invasive surgeries that typically happen between nine and eleven months of age come from the cutting of bone. The more bone to cut, the more bleeding and blood loss, but the children have left far behind their physiologic nadir and therefore the risk of anemia lessens.

For both types of surgery, the anesthesia is distributed based on weight (kilos), and this must be, as Dr. Jeffreys noted, precisely measured, because with children there is no room for error with dosage.

There are times, rough times, when families have dealt with all the waiting and the surgery day comes, but because a cold or the flu or random fever that could have never been predicted pops up on the day of surgery or even the day before surgery the surgery must be canceled.

Parents are sometimes furious because the surgery was canceled. They had waited the long hours, prepped their families and friends, and, sometimes, restructured their lives for the necessary prep, travel, and hospital stay that a major surgery like those to release the sutures of a child with craniosynostosis requires.

Sometimes the anesthesiologist must walk out and tell the parents, "I'm sorry, but we have to reschedule." And this rescheduling, for the most part, can't be done within days but must be put on the calendar months away to work with the hospital, the surgeon, the family's schedule, and, most important, the sickness itself. It can be heartbreaking, disappointing, and, yes, sometimes infuriating for parents. We understand why: the buildup, the fear, the strength to take the child to the hospital that day, and then the letdown, like a balloon losing its air or a world-class athlete faltering at the start line of the Olympics—completely draining, emotionally and physically.

But Dr. Nicole Jeffreys, a specialist who deals specifically with infants and children and, many times, with children with craniosynostosis, knows what she is talking about when she answers the question "Why do we have to reschedule?" She's seen frustrated families. She's had to tell families who had traveled from not only other parts of the country but other parts of the world for surgical treatment at Primary Children's that because a flu bug caught their little one they would have to reschedule for another time.

Dr. Jeffreys is not only a specialist and a pediatric anesthesiologist but also a close friend of mine, someone I have known since our middle school years, so when she looked at me across the table at a coffee shop in downtown Salt Lake City and told me it was a very hard thing to do to tell a family who had traveled from Mexico, saved money to get there, and struggled with everything that entailed that their child could not have surgery because of the flu, I believed her.

But I also believe her when she says it's not worth the risk. Her eyes tell me that. And in them I see the levelheadedness of a doctor not willing to risk the life of an infant prevailing over the kindheartedness of a friend who would rather not break a family's heart and would proceed with a risky surgery because of a fever.

I've talked with families who have had to have their surgeries rescheduled, and they were not happy, believing that the fever was used as a bureaucratic fail-safe or technicality, but talking with Dr. Jeffreys that day at the coffee shop, I realized that couldn't be further from the truth.

Anesthesia is very safe. But when small children have a fever greater than 101.3 degrees, a respiratory tract infection, bronchiolitis, croup, or anything of that nature, doctors have to cancel surgery for four to six week because the children are at risk for respiratory problems under anesthesia after surgery. They have smaller airways as it is. They're at a much higher risk if the sickness is located anywhere below the head. If they're getting sick, you don't want them to be recovering from surgery with pneumonia or another respiratory tract sickness.

The hard part is that young children, especially if they have older siblings or are in day care, get sick a lot, so it takes four to six weeks to get over any respiratory problems. It is very difficult to get back into the window of a healthy child, so there are more cancellations in pediatrics than in the adult population.

A child could end up in ICU with a breathing tube or pneumonia or even die (although this risk is very small, it has to be accounted for). It's low, but you can't take that risk. Many parents struggle with the eating guidelines as well, and the surgery must be postponed because the child ate or drank outside those guidelines. It's very difficult to have your child hungry or not having anything to eat by mouth, but during surgery anything can end up in their lungs and that can be extremely dangerous.

"Beat by beat by beat," Dr. Nicole Jeffreys says. These doctors are the ones watching the children. Before and during the surgery.

The Noose

I've only tried to hang myself once. And I know now, like I knew then, that it was a mistake.

At the age of five or six—old enough to remember the scene clearly but still insurmountably stupid—I watched my older brother, Jake, and my cousin Judd tie a thick rope around a tall, thick tree in my grandma's backyard. The tree was as much a part of my childhood as many of my cousins. We had used it for tree houses and monkey bars and sniper perches, and it had been scribbled into the chronicles of family folklore because of the time my dad and uncle Randy piled ten kids, all under the age of ten, onto a tire swing that hung from its sturdiest branch, pushed the swing back and forth between them until the tire—and the screaming children—swung fifteen feet into the air and parallel to the ground, and listened to the sounds of the women on the porch screaming when the rope snapped and the tire and its passengers flew across the yard, slammed to the ground, and rolled twenty feet, cries erupting from the children on the grassy tarmac.

On the gallows day, Jake threw a rope up to Judd, who straddled the same sturdy branch that held the tire swing. Judd tied it around the branch, tugged on it to make sure it wouldn't snap, and slid down the rope to the ground. Together they tied a loop into the rope at the bottom and tugged on it to make sure the knot wouldn't release. When it was secured, Jake climbed the tree trunk, stepping on a torn-up piece of wood for a step that had been nailed to the tree trunk years before, and when the house was sold thirty years later the two-by-four still hung from the trunk, two rusty nails sticking through it. When he got to the wide base of the tree branch at the top of the trunk, Judd swung the rope up to him. Jake climbed up on a higher branch and put his feet into the loop at the end of the rope. He yelled some form of victory cry and swung down off the tree, hooting and howling throughout the ride. The two of them took turns riding the rope swing, pushing me out of the way and telling me that I was too young to ride on it. When they got tired of it, they headed out into the fields behind my grandma's house to do something they weren't supposed to do.

I stood at the base of the tree alone and stared at the rope swing. With my brother and cousin gone, I had my shot to try it out, so I hooked the rope around my right arm and carried it up the one stair to the top of the tree trunk. I put my foot in the loop and looked down. The distance to the ground scared me. If I had put my foot in and swung from that point, I would have been way too far off the ground for my own comfort. In my young mind, I realized that if I put the rope around my neck and swung from the tree, my feet would be much closer to the ground, and I would have much less space to fall if the rope snapped like it did with the tire swing, so I wrapped the rope around my neck, let go, and swung from the tree branch.

The rope snapped tight above me. The wind came out of my lungs. I dangled there for a few seconds until I heard my grandma scream from her kitchen window when she saw her grandson swinging in the afternoon breeze. My world went black. When I woke up, Grandma had me in her arms and rubbed lotion on a one-inch-thick rope burn that ran from my right ear, down beneath my jawline, and back up to my left ear. The burn, red and black and leaking puss, stayed thick and gross for weeks that summer. In grocery stores, at the movies, and in restaurants, my mom voluntarily told people that I tried to swing from a rope with my neck and watched people's faces as they looked at her as if she were being dumb or rudely euphemistic.

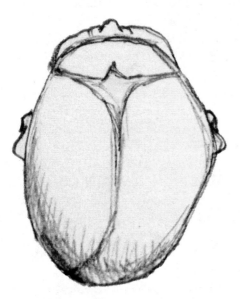

The skull with lambdoid synostosis (courtesy of Sean Davis).

* * *

I don't remember the cut of the spinning blade that sliced through my skull or the blood and the cries and the crack of bone when the saw had done its job. There is, of course, a scar that runs from the crown of my head to my forehead. But, in truth, the pink line of long-ago-coagulated blood has only hurt my sense of vanity. To my mom, however, the slicing into my skull left a scar that runs so deeply through her soul that she still elbows my father in the ribs when the subject of my birth defect or the surgery comes up and makes him talk about it. That bloody memory never coagulated in her. It still runs wet and moist and red and thick.

I always wanted a buzz cut or a flattop or to shave my head completely. Every summer, my older brother would walk into my parents' bathroom and walk out ten minutes later with a fuzzy head, his hair standing an eighth of an inch off his scalp. He'd run around all summer with no hair, freeing him to feel the cool stream of water when we swam in the deep pools of the Weber River and the breeze beneath his baseball cap. His tan ran from his round head to his feet, and when his hair grew back he'd walk back into my parents' bathroom and walk back out fuzzy again.

It may have been my eternal desire to be exactly like my older brother or my internal need to feel like I wasn't different that made me envy the freedom of being hairless for three months of the year, but either way, the freedom was not mine to have.

"Why can't we shave my head?" I asked my mom. I stood at the edge of the bathroom and watched my brother's hair fall to the ground in chunk after chunk. He'd look at me from the corners of his eyes and tell me that I couldn't get my head shaved because I would look like Frankenstein. His eyes would roll back toward the floor and watch the rest of his seasonal locks fall to the ground.

"Quiet, Jake," my mom would say. "It's because of your scars, sweetheart." She'd continue to buzz the hair along the edge of Jake's ears. "I'm sorry." Her guilt showed in her face in the shape of downturned lips and briefly closed eyes and a long inhale and exhale, as if she were breathing in the memory for a moment, closing her eyes to keep her pain and love for her infant son real, and then exhaling to let it go into the world.

Without fail, I walked to the mirror, dropped my head down enough to see the crown of my head and used my fingers to split my dirty blond hair down the middle. With my head down, I could barely see anything, so I would tell my mom that it didn't look that bad and that I would happily climb into the chair next, even going to the point of grabbing a towel beneath the sink and throwing it around my neck to match my brother's towel that, by that time, had become drenched in hair and sweat.

Without fail, my mom would grab a round hand mirror and hold it behind me and split my hair with her fingers. The bathroom mirror reflected what the round mirror reflected—a giant scar that consumed the center of my skull.

"I love you, sweetheart," she said. "If you want me to shave it, I will." She meant it. She would do anything to make me happy.

"I wouldn't. You'll look creepy," my brother said. For a ten-year-old boy giving his brother advice, it was probably the best he could do.

With the mirror above my head, with my brother's words in my mind, and with my thorough knowledge of how cruel children can be, I decided to not get buzzed for another summer. The next time I saw all of my older male cousins, all of them had buzzed heads, a tradition started years ago by my mom and aunts to lessen the trouble of cleanliness. Their boys spent every summer day swinging into the river, climbing in trees, and wrestling in any mud puddle they could find. Less hair meant less dirt.

A buzz cut, not being able to have one, began a hated relationship between my hair, my scalp, and the birth defect that gave the hatred to me.

In fifth grade, at St. Joseph Elementary School, flattops were all the rage. Screen icons like Arnold Schwarzenegger and Val Kilmer and Kurt Russell and Tom Cruise saved the country and got the women; they all wore flattops. One day, it seemed, every kid in class wanted a flattop. They wanted their hair to stick exactly one inch off their heads to match Jean-Claude Van Damme's. Those weeks, it seemed, half of the class came to school with that exact look. Unable to escape the pull of conformism, I wanted one too.

The next day, I sat in a salon chair at John's Salon. Pictures of models with flashy hairstyles were taped on the mirror. The smell of hair products and cigarette smoke sat in the air, and Big John spun me around in the chair, wrapped the cape around my neck, and sat back comfortably in his cushy red vinyl chair. He smoked one last drag from his cigarette, crushed the ashes in his ashtray, and asked me what I wanted to do with my hair.

It felt cool to be asked such a grown-up question, like God had given me some influence on my own personality or my brother had asked me which end of a candy bar I would like to eat.

"You can look at some of these magazines if you'd like while I prep your head," Big John, my stylist, said.

I skimmed through the magazines until I found a section with male models wearing trendy hairstyles of the mid–1980s, mostly replicas of the Cure hairstyles. Nowhere in there was Jean-Claude Van Damme or Arnold Schwarzenegger, so I put the magazine down and leaned in to tell him exactly what I wanted.

"I want a flattop," I told Big John.

John had cut my mom's hair for years, and she had begun taking us there after we could no longer survive in the private school climate with buzz cuts and, for me, bowl cuts. John was big. His belly stuck out a foot from his waist and began just beneath his chest and ended near his knees. To cut hair, he needed to lean on to his belly and rest his elbow on his gut. He hid his face behind a giant beard. To be honest, knowing my mom, I was surprised she let this burly, fat man touch her, but he was good at what he did.

My mom told John about my scar, so he placed his hand on my scalp and gently ran his fingers beneath my hair, letting the bumps and scars raise and lower his fingers until he placed all ten of his fingers on my head, squeezed tightly, and said, "I can't do it." Beneath his beard, his lips, the only visible part of his face beside his eyes and upper cheekbones, scrunched up in what I believe was disappointment in himself, his inability to do what a customer had asked him to do, like a proud samurai laying down his sword made of plastic bristles.

"I can make it stick straight up like a flattop," he said, "but any shorter than four inches and your scar will poke out."

"Okay," I said. All I heard was him say was "stick straight up," and that sounded like a flattop to me. "Let's go for it!" I'd become so excited that I began imagining my flattop at school, girls talking about how cool I was because I had a flattop like Jean-Claude Van Damme, and I began to plan a strict stretching routine so I could do the splits over the edges of two chairs like Van Damme did in the movie *Blood Sport*.

John lifted my hair between his fingers and snipped off the strands that stuck out through the tops of his fingers. A little bit of hair fell to the ground, but as I watched the thin wisps of my dirty blond hair fall, even as a dumb fifth grader I knew that Big John was not cutting enough off to give me a flattop, and I was mad about it. My eyes scrunched, and I looked at my mom in the mirror. She avoided complete eye contact with me while she flipped through the pages of a hairstyle magazine, her version of the whistling bystander.

Then, as if not cutting my hair at all, he put his scissors down. My hair fell down the sides of my head and looked not much different than when I had gotten there, except for all the hair on the top of my head lay at exactly the same length.

"Now, let's style it," Big John said. His breath smelled like the ass of a dead cat.

Style it? I thought. *How about we cut it into a flattop first?*

John rolled his lazy self across the floor, using his chair as a vehicle to grab some styling gel and hair spray. Then he rolled back and placed his forearms on his belly, spun me away from the mirror, and with a comb raised my hair in the air and sprayed it with a tidal wave of aerosol hair spray. His breath mixed with the heavy aerosol smell, and I imagined whatever he ate for lunch getting stuck in my hair for life.

When he was done, when he finally stopped lifting and spraying, he spun me around to the mirror again.

"There we go," he said.

My mom glanced up at my head in the mirror. She saw my wide-open eyes.

"I'll go pay," she said. She gave me a thumbs-up in the mirror and walked toward the reception desk to pay for my flattop without saying another word.

In the mirror sat a young man who looked like he had spent his entire morning rubbing a balloon across his head and when every hair stood up he sprayed his head with transparent glue. I looked more like a porcupine than an action hero. The sides of my head looked like normal dry hair, but the four-inch-high mass of hair that stood up on the top of my head looked wet and gooey.

I started to lose my hair during my senior year of high school, and by the time I started my freshman year of college I had begun to part my hair slightly farther down the side of my head to cover my receding hairline. Every time I showered, hair built up so thick around the drain that I had to pry the silver plug off the top and push the hair down with a hanger I kept by the shower. Going bald at nineteen years old will shock the confidence of any young man. It will make him shy away from women, even if that is something he had never done before. It will make him wear hats more days than not. It will make him let go of his body because he will think there is no reason to keep it in shape. With each hair that falls out, more self-confidence falls—this is for any young man. But I feared more than all of this. At the top of my forehead sat a deep pink scar, nearly half an inch wide and six inches long. It began at my forehead and weaved its way through a landscape of bumps until it stopped at the edge of my frontal hairline. With each strand of hair that fell to the shower basin I feared that my Frankenstein head would be revealed.

Each morning before class, I stood in the mirror and prayed that no more hair would fall from the front or the back of my head, but my prayers were not answered—the balding not only continued through the end of my first semester in college but also sped up, and I began covering my head with a hat that I had borrowed from my roommate, a hat that fell so far down around all edges of my head that it still looked like I had a full head of hair.

I wondered if the balding might stop, but my wondering ended as quickly as it began. The men on my mom's side of the family, my grandfather and uncle, had very little hair on the top of their heads, and some of my older cousins struggled to cover up their balding right alongside me. The heredity war had been fought, and the Cordovan hair follicles had lost the battle. The balding would not stop. It would keep coming until it revealed the ugliness that lay beneath my thinning hair.

My parents noticed it too. And it was due to their guilt and notice of my worry and my stress—not theirs—that they suggested a hair transplant to protect me, again. Deep down, even though they would never admit it, they felt like they had done something that contributed to my craniosynostosis. They didn't take drugs, my mom had never been a drinker, but they felt that if they didn't mix their specific genes my sutures wouldn't have closed early, a worry that affects so many families.

My father's mentor at the time, Bob, a rich man with diamonds on his fingers the size of gobstopper candies, had covered his bald head with plugs the size of nickels. My parents told me they would pay for it if I wanted to go that route. I didn't want to. I saw what Bob's head looked like. His hair plugs were like the Great Wall of China—they could be seen from the moon. Being a kid with a large pink scar and a lumpy head would be better than being a twenty-year-old kid with hair plugs. There was no way I was going to look like a sixty-five-year-old man who couldn't let go of his youth, but after some talking my parents convinced me to visit my aunt and uncle in California and get a consultation from a plastic surgeon. The doctor showed me that Bob's implants were old school, that my implants would be unnoticeable, and that it would be best to do it then because he could plant them next to all the rest of my follicles and no one would know because he wouldn't alter my hairline and it wouldn't look like hair came out of nowhere overnight.

My parents wavered on this decision. They told me how handsome I was. They told me that the right woman wouldn't care about the scars. In a way, I believe they wished they had never brought up the option because, in the end, they really didn't want me to go through with it. But once the option was there, I couldn't get it out of my mind, and I pushed them to fulfill the request.

I got the transplant three weeks later over Christmas break with the hope that by the time spring semester started I would be healed. It was all my decision. I flew to California and lay down on the doctor's table, and with a laser he cut a deep line of hair from ear to ear from the back of my head just above the neck and plugged the hairs into my scalp along the edge of my scar. Then I flew home.

In order for the newly created scar on the back of head to heal (a scar nearly as large as the one on the top of my head), I had to massage a thick layer of Neosporin into my hair and onto my scalp. The gooiness of it saturated my entire head, and not wanting to look like a greaser from the fifties, I walked into Christmas Eve Mass with a hat on and Neosporin, thinned by sweat, dripped down the back of my neck.

Old women tapped me on my shoulder and told me it was disrespectful to wear my hat in Mass. Friends from college and high school stared at the greasiness that lined the edge of my hair, and the paranoia that everyone knew what I had done made the Neosporin more viscous with nervous sweat. I walked from my seat and into the men's bathroom fifteen minutes into Mass and didn't leave until the church had cleared out, avoiding all the friends and families who usually hung out after Mass to talk, catch up, and laugh. I sat with my head in my hands and let the sticky flow of liquid from my head pool up in puddles on the bathroom floor. I hated my head. I hated that I had cosmetic surgery to cover it up. I hated that I looked like a disrespectful punk in mass. I hated that I knew I would lie about my transplant for the rest of my life. I hated that I wasn't braver.

Like only trying to hang myself once, I've only really had my heart broken once—in my adult life at least, as we have all had the many broken crushes of youth. After a study abroad trip in 1997 to Mexico, where I spent the whole time living like I believed a twenty-one-year-old boy should live in Mexico, bouncing from bar to bar and futbal match to futbal match and staying out way to late, I felt like I needed to grow up, to get a real girlfriend, and to become an adult—this feeling of wanting to become a man my father would be proud of, a strong man, still pulls on me today even though I have a beautiful wife, a brilliant son, and a great job. This feeling of never grasping manhood scares me. It makes me wonder if I will ever know myself or own who I have become or, more important, who I have always been.

A good friend of mine at work set me up with a mature girl, someone with her head on her shoulders, someone who knew what she wanted in life. She planned to graduate early from college, had never partied in her life, and was a strict Mormon. Growing up in Utah, I told myself I would never date Mormons, but my work friend assured me that this girl was different and she wouldn't care about my conversion. So I went out on the date, not really expecting anything but a nice afternoon in the foothills of the Rocky Mountains.

On our first date, we stood at the bottom of the trailhead at North Fork Canyon in northern Utah. It was the perfect date because I was nervous and we didn't need to talk. At the trailhead, we exchanged glances....

Writing down the details of the relationship is unnecessary. It followed the path of most failed college relationships. It rose and fell through fun times, awful times, and awkward times. At one point she felt more for me, and at another time I felt more for her—this shifted the power toward the one who cared least at the moment, as it does with most relationships. Then, one morning in the spring of 1998, I walked out to my Jeep to go to class and found a note tucked under the windshield wiper on the driver's side.

"You're not who you used to be, it's time we broke up. Please don't call or come by. This is final," the note read. At that time, obviously, she was the one who cared least and I was the one who cared most. I crumpled the note in my hand, walked back into the house, took off my clothes, and climbed into bed. I didn't leave the comfort of my covers until the next morning.

I thought about her a lot and was dumbfounded by how hard the breakup had hit me. I hadn't felt that torn up since my high school girlfriend went to college in another state, and even then I got over the breakup much more quickly. The toughest part to understand was that I really couldn't pin down why I missed her so much. We shared few common interests. We weren't active sexually. She hated it when I drank and hung out with my friends. And, many times I had to have a couple drinks with my buddies to hang out with her. We were not meant to be together. I knew that from the beginning, but I was still heartbroken and thought about her every day for months after the breakup. It's something I can only admit now.

But the breakup note or losing her would only be a prologue to how deeply she cut me. One night, after going to the bar with friends, I couldn't stop thinking about her. My friends and I sat on our deck, drank beer, and welcomed friends to join us. Having drunk too much already, I did what no guy should do; I started talking about her openly, rambling on about missing her, blabbering on about getting her back. By that time late spring had come and warmed up the days of northern Utah, but at night winds pushed through Ogden Canyon, picked up the mist of the cold Ogden River, and fell like a chilly sheet onto the Ogden valley, so we moved into the house. That's when I headed for the phone—not a cell phone but a plugged-in phone in my room, the common use of cell phones still a couple years in the future.

My evening's previous blabbering about her alerted every close friend in the room. They shouted, "Stop him. He's gonna call her. Stop him now. Kase, you'll regret it tomorrow!" Then, my best friend grabbed both my arms from behind, hoisted me in the air, and pinned me to the ground, using his military training to render me immobile.

"No good will come from that phone call," he said in my ear. The smell of beer and sweat blew past me. "She's no good for you. It's time to stop this shit." He lessened his grip on my arm but kept my face on the ground. All I could see was rebel carpet fiber that shot up from the floor and the shoes of the rest of my friends. Dust rose up from my face slamming into the floor. The world began to spin, and I nearly passed out right then.

"I'll let you up if you promise to not call her," my friend said. He eased his forearm off the back of my neck and brought me up to my knees.

"I swear," I said. He let me go. I was beaten, for the moment.

The night sang on with music and laughter and arguments and cigarette smoke that snuck in through the front door. One by one, anyone who didn't live there with me left, saying good-bye and slamming their beer before walking away, and then my best friend left and my roommates went to sleep.

I was alone again. The room spun around me, and I stumbled into my bedroom. I lowered myself down onto the edge of my bed and picked up the phone receiver. The numbers, while big and bulky, seemed nearly impossible to hit with fingers. The phone swung back and forth in the palm of my hand. The numbers blurred. Time and time again, I messed up the sequence, getting either an error message or a wrong number. Where this type of determination comes from while drinking is unknown. Sober, after one or two tries at something I give up, finding something on TV, looking for food in the fridge, grading a horribly written composition essay. But while drinking at twenty-two years of age I did not give up until I punched in her number and, after I hit redial several times and letting the machine pick it up, she answered.

"Kase, stop calling me. I'm with my boyfriend," she said into the phone.

Most everyone has been there. They believe that if they tell the person who denies their affection that they love them then the person will, although having heard this one hundred times before, magically hang up the phone, drop their new lover, and rush to the arms of their drunken suitor at that exact moment. It's not just saying, "I love you"; it's the belief that if they call late at night and say it with tears in their eyes and yearning in their voice that will do the magic. I felt that way that night with my tears and my yearning. I believed.

"I have something to tell you," I said. My voice cracked and sputtered, and I made sure to sniffle really loudly into the phone to make sure she knew I had been crying or holding back tears. "It's so important." Her boyfriend spoke in the background, and she had become completely silent. A gasp fell from her mouth and onto the receiver, and in my mind I felt like she was ready to hear what I had to say, as if she had been waiting for it and the gasp was her physical signal for me to go ahead.

"I have to tell you something," I said. Breath filled my lungs to release the most powerful "I love you" I had ever released.

But she spoke first. "What? About your hair transplant? I already know. Now leave me alone." The sarcasm and cruelty in her voice pushed the air from my lungs like the tightrope swing nearly twenty years earlier. She knew I was born without soft spots and that a long scar covered my head. She knew I worried about my scars. No, I never told her about my transplant, as I was completely embarrassed by it, but she knew her response was her best noose to hang any of my hopes. And it did.

The Plateau

A railway trench, like a deep and open suture, cut through the limestone mountains of the Castilian plateau in northern Spain. The railway suture opened up earth between the green and brown farmlands of the plateau. Tunnels of limestone hung above the completed track and straight, sharp walls looked down on the workers who moved through the drying Spanish terra until, in the early nineteenth century, they found a series of caves dug out of the earth as if from the hand of a surgeon's scalpel. La Trinchera del Ferrocarril, the trench of the railway line that was never completed, led into the caves, and within them the railway workers found shelters cut into the limestone. The paleokarsts, ancient caves made up of soluble sediment and formed by flowing water—revealed by the cutting of the trinchera—opened up an ancient world of hominins and animals that roamed the earth hundreds of thousands of years ago. For thousands of years, humans walked between the sage only meters above another world where humankind set up shelter away from the dangers on the surface of the earth. The water table that filled the caves dropped and left only clean freshwater at the entrances of the vast and wiggling cave system, which, in turn, made the ancient dwelling exceptional for habitation with protection from the elements and predators as well a clean water source.

Limestone corridors wind through the dura of the earth's crust. Narrow passageways open up into large cathedral-like rooms where giant stalactites hang down tens of feet toward the base of the cave, their growth, deposition of calcium carbonate and other minerals, extending downward at less than a centimeter per year. Light comes in from the cave entrances and cool air flows through the caves, and beneath the sediment lies the most important anthropological digging site in Europe and possibly the entire world. Tools and weapons and drawings were discovered and are still being excavated from the karsts, in the sediment and on the walls of the cave system, but, most important, archeologists found the largest bone deposit of hominins in the world to this date.

In the very southeast corner of the Sala de los Ciclopes, a wide-open cave that spreads outward and upward like the expanse of great concert halls, researchers found a deep pit around seven meters wide and ten meters long. Archeologists had been systematically excavating the pit since 1984. They have found the remains of at least thirty-two hominins at the bottom of the Sima de los Huesos, the largest collection anywhere in the world. After digging and digging, the scientists discovered the lack of herbivores among the fossils at the bottom of the pit, leading them to believe that pit was a burial ground instead of a dwelling place—a mortuary. While scientists disagree about the age of the fossils, they do agree that the fossils are the oldest found in Europe (more than two hundred thousand years old), and that the Sima de los Huesos contains the largest dump of fossils that old, making it the most important dig site in Europe. In 2001 the slow and meticulous excavation discovered a skull not like any of the other skulls that lay on the base of the Sima de los Huesos. The cranial shape, inside and outside of the skull, was gravely deformed. One archeologist leans against the wall of the fossil-rich land; the skull is buried deep in the wall behind, and it sticks only halfway out—its profile visible to the outside world. The skull is nearly fully intact, but unlike the other skulls dug up among the thirty-two hundred pieces of fossils of hominins, this skull, from the frontal view, has a left temporal bone and left eye socket that drop way beneath those of its right side. Looking from above, the straight, vertical forehead is drastic and shockingly straight and the bulging and swelling of the skull above the eye cannot be mistaken for normal growth in a human skull, and from the inside of the skull, the deformities are even more traumatic, as the cranium is squeezed and pulled toward the left of the "sagittal plane." All of these deformities of the skull led anthropologists to the conclusion that this skull belonged to a hominin, born hundreds of thousands of years ago, with lambdoid synostosis, the rarest of the five major sutures that break up the major bones of the cranium.

Cranium 14 told the anthropologists a lot, as it should tell those who either were born with craniosynostosis or have children who were born with craniosynostosis. First, the pathology of single suture craniosynostosis has been part of our history, even though very rare, for hundreds of thousands of years. The extent of the abnormalities in Cranium 14, an immature adult as scientists believe, and the severity of the abnormalities at death show that the defect developed before the child's birth, like most who develop craniosynostosis today. Also, the severity of the misshapenness of the head led researchers to believe that the immature adult suffered "motor and cognitive" disorders that were onset because of lambdoid single suture synostosis, the brain finding it difficult to grow where it needed to grow with the cranial shape described previously. It also tells us that those with whom the immature adult lived with were, as some authors and paleoanthropologists suggest, a caring group in her society, since Cranium 14 had lived into young adulthood and would have needed extra care from the prehistoric community to do so, understanding that with motor and cognitive disabilities the child would not be able to survive on her own and would take away food from healthy children in the society.

Cranium 14, at the end of her life, was tossed down into the burial shaft of La Sima de los Heusos along with at least thirty-two others from her community. She lived a short life, relative to ours, and she had no option of release of her lambdoid suture. Today, nearly half a million years later, the ossification of the lambdoid suture, occurring in 2 to 3 percent of children born with craniosynostosis, can be released through both the use of a full vault and endoscopic procedures and these procedures follow the same success and failure patterns as the other surgical release of the other single suture synostosis. The diagnosis of the lambdoid suture, like the others, has its own hiccups. While the metopic suture craniosynostosis diagnosis is gray because of the early closure of the suture and need for surgery and the sagittal suture synostosis is sometimes brushed aside as coming about because of a difficult birth, the closing of the lambdoid suture is commonly mistaken as positional plagiocephaly and vice versa.

Positional plagiocephaly is common among infants and recognizable by the flatness of the infant's head on one side or the other in the back or front. Deformational plagiocephaly can occur because of lack of growth in the womb due to many different factors, such as lack of oxygen to the fetus, poor nutritional habits of the mother, and, sometimes, the mother's prescription use during pregnancy; birthing position, how the baby came out of the womb; or back sleeping. Typically, deformational plagiocephaly is symmetrical in its deformation; for instance, if the right back side of the infant's head has flattened, the right front side of the infant's head protrudes forward, the left back of the head bosses and the left front side moves backward toward the bossing. All of this movement in the skull compensates for the flattening of the back right side of the skull and leaving room for the brain to grow without high ICP (increased cranial pressure). It's like holding a bag of rice in your hand and pushing the right side forward while pulling the left side back. The rice follows the sack forward on the right-hand side and backward on the left with no less space within the bag. There is no real bulge in the bag, just shifting of the allotted space. With true lambdoid synostosis, however, the skull does not compensate symmetrically.

A lambdoid suture pulls everything to one side when it is closed. Since the suture is closed, there will be no movement among the adjacent skull bones; therefore, they can't shift forward to compensate for the fused suture. Typically, this results in a flattening of the affected side and a bulging of the other side along with enlargement over the eye of the opposite side. On the affected side, the forehead, eye, and ear are pulled backward toward the fused suture, unlike deformational plagiocephaly, where they move forward to compensate for the flattening in the back. Imagine that same bag of rice. With true lambdoid synostosis, one side of the bag of rice is pinched and immovable. The rice then pushes to the opposite side and is squished against the bag and creates pressure between the rice and bag and bulges out on the nonaffected side and pulls to the pinched area on the affected side. While there are, of course, exceptions to the generalized difference between the two deformations, this deformational difference can usually distinguish between the two prior to other types of medical diagnosis options like X-ray and CT scans, which many craniofacial specialists do not use.

While treatment of plagiocephaly does not call for surgery, it still must be treated or the problem with the skull can persist. Helmet therapy for moderate to severe cases does not just reposition the bones in the skull but reshapes them as well. The helmet, most important, ensures that the child does not lie on the affected side and this protection allows the brain and skull to grow. Research suggests that the sooner the better when it comes to helmet therapy for children with positional plagiocephaly. The sooner-the-better option yields faster and, typically, better results, with four to six months the optimum range. Most doctors believe and have shown through their research that there is no risk in developmental disabilities in children with treated and untreated positional plagiocephaly because the skull, since the sutures are not closed, allows the bones to shift backward and forward without creating pressure on the brain. But getting the diagnosis correct is very important, as research shows that children with single suture synostosis, in this case lambdoid synostosis, do run 10 to 15 percent elevated developmental risk without corrective surgery (and some studies suggest the percent of elevated risk is much higher).

The lambdoid suture must be released. One major study produced by J.M. Smart, Jr., and his team of plastic surgeons confirmed much of the previously stated research. They studied children at the Children's Hospital of Philadelphia (CHOP) between the years 1990 and 2005. Unlike the families of children born with sagittal single suture synostosis or metopic single suture synostosis, few families walked into CHOP with a child whose lambdoid suture had closed. The surgeons looked at placement and symmetry of facial features, as well as scans. They followed nine patients. Six of the children underwent corrective surgery and three did not. The surgeons weren't able to collect data on developmental or cognitive disabilities, but they were able to take an objective look at physical symmetry of the facial features of the children. Across the board, there was not one specific consistent facial asymmetry in those children who did not have corrective surgery, but there was one consistency among them: the three who did not have corrective surgery had a very noticeable asymmetry of the face or a combination of asymmetries; there was occipital flattening (flattening of the back of the skull), bulging of either the affected or unaffected side, and a major deficiency of the facial bones on the unaffected side of the face. Those who received the cranioplasty in the first year of their lives were able to avoid any of the previously mentioned asymmetries.

In the hills of Atapuerca, beneath the dura of the earth, scientists dug up a skull with lambdoid synostosis. The rich brown earth kept it nearly whole while hundreds of thousands of years passed by above on the earth's surface. Through all that time, children were born with the premature ossification of their lambdoid suture (or any other suture for that matter) without the opportunity to have it surgically corrected, but within the last forty to sixty years of human existence surgeons have opened up opportunities of a normal life that Cranium 14 couldn't have in the primitive life she lived hundreds of thousands of years ago. Like a suture that runs through the skull, the railroad trench released the secrets of the past into the hands of scientists. Those secrets revealed that craniosynostosis, even in its rarest form, has been with us from the beginning. The pathoanthropology of the birth defect should give those parents who believe they did something wrong some release from their guilt. The birth defect is a birth defect is a birth defect, void of guilt or shame or time—predominantly. Cranium 14 showed us that.

PART FOUR: THE CROWN
(CORONAL SYNOSTOSIS)

Intruder

I felt like an intruder and, more than that, a very late intruder when I threw the door open to the lobby of the hotel and shook Jennifer's hand and gave a little wave to Kaiya, an infant with right unilateral coronal craniosynostosis. Google Maps had told me their hotel was right next to mine in North Dallas, so I had left with five minutes to get there, nearly forty-five minutes earlier, and had spent the last forty minutes flying around corners in North Dallas and sweating and cussing and talking to Jennifer on the phone as she relayed the front desk worker's directions across the line.

Ten minutes before I walked into, rushed and covered in sweat, the hotel lobby, I almost gave up, called Jennifer, apologized profusely for making her wait for me, and drove away home to Manhattan, Kansas, full of guilt and anger and frustration and regret. I didn't want her to wait in a hotel lobby for me any longer. Jennifer and Kaiya were in North Dallas to have Kaiya's suture released and skull resculpted, and it was obvious that I was there to meet them. But the longer I drove around, sweat starting to pour out of me even though the air-conditioned car was full of frigid air, the more I worried about Jennifer more than anything else. Kaiya had no real idea what was coming in two days; she would never remember the trip to Dallas and would never remember the lobby of a hotel in North Dallas or waiting for what seemed to be a flaky writer, even though I am usually one those highly punctual freaks.

Jennifer had just a few hours with her baby girl before she would be taken away. Though surgery for craniosynostosis has become very safe, the fear of losing her forever to complications, blood loss, or any other of the problems that cause the very small percentage of loss of life during infant surgery was very real— and it doesn't matter how small the percentage is; to those families who lose a child under the knife, the loss of life is 100 percent, and I couldn't stop thinking about that and how, with every minute, I ate into that precious time alone.

I felt like an intruder when I finally walked into the hotel lobby, a thief stealing precious minutes from Jennifer and her baby, a pirate looting the treasure of time from a mother whose face gave me a look, even if she didn't mean to and even if she was warm and nice, that told me as much. She led me to a table where she had set up Kaiya's high chair and had been feeding her snacks. I sat, opened my briefcase, and pulled out my microphone and recorder and set it up as quickly as I could, my mind spinning with insecurities about what the hell I thought I was doing there with this family, who the hell did I think I was invading their privacy and asking them questions about "how they felt" right then before surgery. Wouldn't that be obvious? Wouldn't the fear and worry and doubts that I had encountered in previous interviews, relayed to me post-op from parents on the other side, be enough to fill in the gaps? Did this woman hate me for asking for the interview and for being late? Why couldn't I just fill in the gaps on my own?

But it was different to sit with Jennifer two days before the surgery, much different from listening to parents try to recall their feelings and emotions from a time when most of them mostly talked about living in a haze of numbness and fear. That numbing fear sat in front of me that hot Dallas morning. Kaiya ate her snacks. The custodial staff ran a loud vacuum behind us. The hotel AC kicked on loud to beat away the Texas heat that would try to infiltrate the lobby that day, and when I got started with questions I felt like an invasive fraud, although I had done interviews for years.

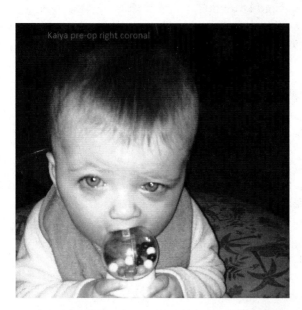

Kaiya pre-op right coronal

Photograph of Kaiya pre–surgery for unilateral coronal craniosynostosis (courtesy of Jennifer McFarland).

"So, tell me about Kaiya," I said.

Guarded, taken aback, Jennifer started by running her hands over Kaiya's head and over her left brow that fell over her eye. The bone hung there like a rock above a cliff on the edge of the sea of Kaiya's bright, bright blue eyes. Her forehead, very typical for unilateral coronal craniosynostosis, fell from the unaffected side to the affected side like someone was pulling down on that side of her head. The right coronal suture closed early, forbidding it to expand, pushing her brain backward and sideways toward the part of her skull that could grow and pulling her sutureless plate downward. Her right eye, beautiful in all its blueness, shone brightly as she looked at her mom, and her left eye, still blue and bright, hid a bit beneath that part of the skull that was doing its best to grow in any way that it could.

"Hmm," Jennifer started. "What do you want to know?" She is guarded, she leans backward away from me, and there is no hint of a smile on her lips, but *why should there be?* I ask myself. Again I felt the fraud and the intruder. I was there to write a book about her experience, and I wanted a smile that morning two days before surgery? She squinted at me, her eyelids tight against her pupils, gauging if she could trust this man in front of her. When she wasn't feeding Kaiya in those longer-than-life minutes, Jennifer's hands were squeezed together and she sighed deeply, her breath leaving her and carrying her worries outward into the world, but until the surgery was complete no amount of exhales could purge her of her fears, and I had the gall to ask her to talk about it. I would ask a few more questions over the next fifteen minutes, but I knew, even though Jennifer was more than kind and forgiving of my tardiness, that they had the day planned together in the last few hours before surgery. I said, "Good luck," and wondered if by saying "good luck" I might sound like there was a chance bad luck could rear its ugly head and there might be major complications that could even result in death, so I followed it up with an "it will all be fine" but scrambled in my head to cover that one up, as it might seem like I thought what they were going through and would go through in the upcoming weeks was small, trivial, and common.

Talking to a parent who is at the brink of handing her child over before major surgery was hard, and it was something that I'd never done before, so I stumbled around with my words, knowing that whatever I said could negatively affect the mother in front of me, add worry to an already-overbearing world of worry, or even just plant a seed in her mind that she had effectively already ripped out and tossed away from her conscious thoughts in the interest of self-preservation. God didn't come up in our brief conversations, and this is a tricky one for all of us who roam this planet, so I said my thoughts would be with her and her family, shook her hand, said, "Thank you," and turned to walk away.

"Well, in a week this will all be over," she said, her words following me as I turned toward the door.

Jennifer talked about how her second child had mild metopic, how they had met with the doctors, and how the doctors had decided to not operate on her, to Jennifer and her husband's relief. When Kaiya was born, they didn't notice the flattening of the right side of her head, saw her as the most beautiful of babies, her bright blues shining out at the world, but then the right side flattened, making her left eye appear less open than her right eye. Then the worries came, and at that point in the story, Jennifer stopped talking, closed up again.

The day before the interview, she took Kaiya to the doctor's office. The anthropologist took more than one hundred measurements of Kaiya's head by wrapping his hands around her gently enough to keep her from being upset. From there, they were shuttled to the media department of the craniofacial center, where the photographer snapped fifteen to twenty photos of Kaiya from many different perspectives around her—these may pop up someday as before and after photos on the craniofacial center Web site for awareness or for before and after success and, yes, maybe for promotion. Kaiya, passed between anthropologist and media, was tired, having just flown with her family from Ohio the night before, but she remained smiley throughout the first part of the extensive check-in day, but then the fun stopped. Two pricks to the scalp and one to the foot to draw blood for vitals brought out the screams of the little girl.

"That was not fun. They had to take a lot of blood upstairs for vitals," Jennifer said. She paused and looked at her little girl, who swiped her snacks from the plastic surface of her chair.

"The geneticist basically cleared her of a syndrome. That was a relief," Jennifer said. Then, in almost a daze, she continued. Their plastic surgeon, Dr. Fearon, came in and talked to them. He calmed their nerves enough to make it through the evening and through the weekend, except that calming feeling in the surgeon's office wore off before Friday night had ended.

On Monday morning at 7:45, Jennifer and her husband, Ray, handed Kaiya over. They cried in the elevator as it dropped down floor by floor to the general waiting room where their waiting would begin.

"The waiting sucks!" Jennifer said.

* * *

Surgeons, as they all do things just a little differently, will decide which surgical approach to take to release the coronal or bicoronal fusion. Many will use the bitemporal approach, meaning that they will not take off the entire skull from the brow line up and all the way around, but instead they will, generally and depending on the severity of the effects of the fused suture, take off "just" the front half of the skull from the brow up and from the front of the ears forward. This approach—and the following is a summary of the technique—leaves the posterior skull untouched and reveals the forehead, the fused coronal suture, the anterior cranial vault, and a large portion of the facial bones. By removing this part of the skin, surgeons have access to the entire calvarial vault, the front and side skull bases, the frontal sinuses, and the eye and all the bones that surround it. Because the surgery aims to open up the front part of the skull, the incision can be made anywhere near the midline of the skull. The hair around the future point of incision is shaved and the scalp is cleaned. All the necessary steps are taken to ensure the least amount of blood loss during the surgery. Some surgeons use cautery scalpels and others use hemostatic clips, while many use a vasoconstrictor (anything that can narrow the opening of a blood vessel). Compared to years past, blood loss has been decreased significantly and the many techniques are very successful. Surgeons will then elevate the coronal flap to access the fused suture. Fascia (the thick, fibrous connective tissue) is cut. Once the flap has been elevated, surgeons may turn it inside out and let it settle that way, away from the suture, until they are finished. From there, the surgeons will make an incision and lift the pericranial flap (the dense membrane that covers the bone) to expose the skull.

After the incision, the surgeons will cut through numerous layers of tissue and bone, including the skin, the subcutaneous tissues (multiple), and the fascia that surrounds the temporoparietal junction (the meeting between the temporal and parietal bones). In order to access the fused suture and to reconstruct the orbital wall, surgeons, depending on their goals, will expose multiple areas of the bone surrounding those areas to gain access. The surgeons will release the coronal suture, graft bone from other parts of the skull, and reconstruct the anterior skull—the size of the dissection, the amount of grafted bone, and the severity of reconstruction all depend on the child and the preferred surgical technique of the surgeon.

The doctors called Jennifer in after they had performed an extensive CVR—pulling off the skull from the brow line up and breaking it up before placing it back together like a puzzle—on Kaiya. They released the suture, sculpted her eyebrows, and reshaped the entirety of her head to compensate for the lack of growth and future growth of the skull and brain previously dictated by the closed coronal suture.

With Kaiya, and others under the care of Dr. Fearon, all of the surgical repair was done strictly with her own bone and the surgery looked to overcompensate for the continued growth of the little girl. Dr. Fearon explains the reasoning behind the overcompensation of structuring during surgery:

[Overcompensation is] where you take the bone off and you make it actually a larger shape. So in my own practice when I think about what it is we're treating, you know we want. When a suture is fused or shut you get impaired growth in the region of the skull there, but interestingly, the other sutures compensate and they take over and you get more growth of the other sutures. So for each suture that fuses shut there's a combination of a localized impaired growth and an outside beyond that overgrowth to compensate. So it's a good system, and interestingly, the sutures only kind of expand when the brain wants to expand. There's a condition called microcephaly where kids' brains never grow, but we don't find them rattling around inside of bigger skulls that were just growing on their own, so the skull only gets bigger when the brain's trying to enlarge. So if you have a restricted growth in one area it sort of makes sense that the other sutures would take over. And it's probably for this reason that those looking at pressure in the early seventies didn't find elevated pressure in most of the kids they measured, probably because early on those sutures are good at taking the pressure off.

I think later on as the sutures become less critical for skull growth it seems the studies that look at pressure when kids are older are more likely to show high pressures, and I wonder if that's just because the suture's no longer functioning that way and taking them off. That's just speculation.

So, the purpose of the [correction], of any craniosynostosis correction, is to normalize the skull shape and to make sure that the brain can function in a normal way. That's it. And you want to do it with as small and safe an operation as you can. Now, interestingly, we have shown from a lot of studies we've done here that after you do the operation on a child's craniosynostosis as they grow older the skull tends to go back the way it was. Based on that we recommended in publishing our studies that you kind of overcorrect what you see to compensate for that. And the reason that's important is a certain percentage of kids end up getting more than one operation for craniosynostosis, and if it's going back the way it was some older kids, they don't like to have that look and they want another operation. And there've been a few studies that suggest maybe kids even present with signs of raised pressure that had maybe inadequate treatment early on, they're not based on strong science but they're certainly, you know, eye-opening studies.

So one reason kids end up getting second operations is they don't look so good when they're teenagers and the second reason is if the surgeon takes off bone and doesn't replace it or enlarges the skull and there's a gap and doesn't fill it in. When babies are really young they'll fill it in with new bone, but as they get older they're less likely to fill those gaps in. You can overcompensate when you're doing that, you can make it bigger in the directions that you're enlarging because you know it's going to grow back a little bit, and also you have the ability when you take the bone off you can split it like an Oreo cookie and use that extra bone to fill in the gaps that were left by making the skull larger because you take a smaller bowl and you make it bigger you're going to have spaces in between so.

I want to do children just one time, I don't want to do them again, and so I think that gives me the best final result when they're teenagers. But I tell my patients you don't know if you've had a successful operation till your child is a teenager; most parents think if their kid's alive afterwards they've had a successful operation, but it's successful if they look normal and don't have holes in their head when they're sixteen. So the two reasons that kids get second operations are persistent skull defect that's to protect the brain and the other is if the skull shape's gone back so much they don't look normal; they'll tell their parents they want a—they're getting made fun of, they're teased—want another operation.

So when we're trying to decide if we're doing, which operation we're doing, we want to normalize appearance, we want to take the pressure off or improve cerebral blood flow or really prevent neurological problems is the ultimate goal, you want to do it safely and you only want to do one and not have to repeat it. And so ideally surgeons will look at all those different goals and try to decide the best way to do it.

The medical team, confident in their skills, started and finished the CVR (cranial vault remodeling) in only two hours, and Kaiya lay and waited for her mom and dad to pick her up and hold her. When Jennifer first saw her, the swelling had not begun to wrap itself around Kaiya's head. Her doctor, as many doctors chose, did not use any bandages or draining tubes.

"For the first time, the right side of her head wasn't all flat and caved in looking," Jennifer said. "She looked like this is how she was intended to be her whole life."

The first day in the PICU and then the day on the children's recovery floor were very difficult. Kaiya's heart rate jumped and fell, and her swelling came on strong. The little girl became very agitated. She was swollen and unhappy and unable to move and covered in wires to keep her vitals that kept getting pulled off until Jennifer finally took them off herself.

"[Mothers,] BE prepared for vitals to be all over the place in the PICU," Jennifer warns with everything but a whisper. She talks directly to anyone who reads

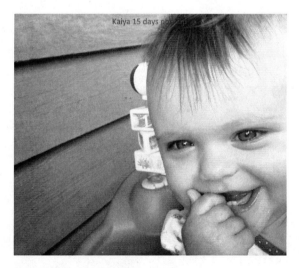

Photograph of Kaiya post–surgery for unilateral coronal craniosynostosis (courtesy of Jennifer McFarland).

this story and who has to experience the same thing. She worries about their feelings when their child's vitals spike and fall and spike and fall again like the jagged waves of music.

By the third day post-surgery, Jennifer held Kaiya in her arms beneath the sunlight of the afternoon. The little girl loved the way the sunlight fell across her face and how its warmth blanketed her in her mother's arms. Kaiya lay in the sunlight in the afternoon until one of her eyes began to open and let in the world again. Then, as if the decrease in the swelling and the opening of the eye were both connected to her tiny mouth, the girl with the beautiful blue eyes started to smile again.

Loosen

The streets of the small Irish town were wet. Micro-streams ran between the cobbles from the high and dark end of the street where we walked to the low end of the street where we were headed, down toward the few lit buildings in the small town in the center of the island. Like a small speck of dust that was picked up on the edges of one of the cobbles and carried without control and without hope of stopping before the end, I walked down the barely lit road in 2001 with a girl I barely knew but a girl I knew I loved. The micro-streams beneath our feet made the streets slick, and I had promised her dinner at a restaurant and not pub fare—I had taken her to pubs every night since she flew into Dublin nearly a week earlier to visit me while I spent the fall writing for the Consumers' Association of Ireland, my post–MA internship. She reached out and grabbed my hand to steady herself. And I grabbed hers back. In the cold fall night in Ireland her hand was warm and soft and her fingers seemed to fall between mine like a tongue meeting a groove. For that brief moment when our hands met, the comfort that she gave me since our first night together a few months earlier during our brief courtship in the Utah summer wiggled its way through and calmed the inevitable cramping that consumed my stomach when I got nervous.

We'd stopped in this random little town on our way back to Dublin that wasn't on our itinerary. When she got off the plane nearly a week earlier, both of us didn't know what the hell we were doing. We'd dated for a month that previous summer and felt like we were in love, but both of us, having dated enough and grown up enough, knew that the first few weeks of any relationship are like flowers, but in time those flowers either wilt away or must fade for winter and then bloom again. We'd both been in relationships that wilted after a few months and then never bloomed again. We'd both also had relationships that bloomed again after a rough, cold, or barren time but sprouted new buds only to have a winter kill them for good, so when she got there, even though we both had fallen heavily for each other in the summer, we knew this week, traveling together across the Irish countryside with no one else around us, with long hours trapped together in a car, and with nothing to do but, intentionally or unintentionally, scratch the surface of our good and bad qualities, would tell us if we should continue a relationship that would need, at the very least, one more year of a long-distance courtship, commitment, and effort. I knew that by the end of that week I had to tell her about my head, about my scars, and about my hair transplant and the plugs on the front of head to hold back the balding that had set in during my late teens.

I knew I had to tell her that night. We would be in Dublin the next night. We would be dealing with saying good-bye. I'd put it off until that point in the trip, telling myself, "This is not the right time. We're having too much fun." I knew it in my gut. If I let her get on that plane two days later without telling her, our trip to know each other would have been a fraud. The night we drove along the five-foot-wide road on the Dingle coast and found a B and B lit up in the middle of complete darkness that looked like the first star in the night against a black sky and in the morning we woke, looked out our window, traced where we had driven the night before, and saw that I had almost driven right off a cliff into the ocean would have been a fraud. The day an ex-girlfriend of mine wrote and told my companion all of our intimate details— she told Mary what I'd said to her during nights of frivolity and drunkenness and that she would be the next in line to hear my lies and eventually be set aside—and I had to explain everything I said in the past and promise that what I had said to her over the summer and the last few nights was the truth, that gut-wrenching afternoon filled with tears and sharp words, would have been a fraud. And the day we sat in Doolin and listened to the Irish band who sang and clattered in the seminal town of Irish folk music and the tourists and the band and the sunlight were nearly nonexistent as we swam in pints of Irish beer and talked about "us." All of these moments of truth would become half-truths if I didn't tell her about the one thing that I had thought about nearly every day of my adult life—I had scars, and I had scars and plugs to cover up scars.

We stopped in front of the only restaurant in the little Irish town. The streetlights shone on the wet cobbles of the road like two pillars of light reaching out to lie on the ground. Three or four pubs were on the street down around a curve of the road, and we stood in front of a Chinese restaurant in the middle of Ireland. I had my doubts about the quality, but I had promised, and I knew that the quiet hum of an empty Chinese restaurant would be a much better place to vomit my worries, insecurities, and vanities onto the table.

Tablecloths of bright red and ornamental pictures and lanterns hung throughout the place when we walked in and asked for a table. We were the only ones there, no music played, and it felt like we were alone for the first time. The awkwardness of silence in a public restaurant sat on us like the heavy clouds sat on the town outside, and, for one of the few times since we'd met, we were quiet.

"What's wrong?" she asked. She didn't beat around the bush and didn't act like the moment, the walk, the night weren't weird. In her mind, we had fought the ex-girlfriend battle and cleared out the demons of the past, and she was happy. I must have seemed odd to her as I sat there tight-lipped and scared, like I had lied to her in the past and now felt those lies cement inside of me.

"Nothing. I just need to eat," I said. Which was true. The swirling pains of worry would be partially calmed with heavy Chinese food.

"Okay?" she said. Then she scanned the menu.

We ordered wine instead of beer for the first time during the trip, and we sipped on it before the waiter came back with our food. The wine buzz, much different from the beer buzz, seeped through me, warming my belly and relaxing my legs.

"So you gonna talk tonight, or are we just going to sit here and look at the menu?" she asked. She giggled a bit and did her best to break the awkward tension that she had no idea why it existed after such a wonderful week filled with smiles and laughter and views from the Irish coast and walks beneath the archways of castles.

"I have to tell you something that I'm not proud of," I said. I sipped from my wine, which had a strong vinegar taste to it, but at the time I thought all wine tasted like that.

"Okay?" she said. She paused for a little bit. "You don't have to." I think that the whole last week flashed before her too and that she didn't want those memories to be lain across the table and diced up. At that moment, I believe she just wanted to live in the goodness that was that week before she had to head back to real life in the states. Her "you don't have to" said it all.

"No, I do," I said. After I had been recently shat on by a girl I loved because I hid my secrets from her, a part of me, right then and right there, along with the need to keep every moment from the last week real, became a little angry and wanted to throw it all out there just to see if it would stick, to see if that cruelty that had stung me in the past would rise up again and sting me again because of my own childish vanity. Part of me was scared to be so heavily in

love with a girl I had only known for four months and of whom my close friend
Heather, whom I had known for decades, who had met her that summer, said,
"She's the one for you. I've met them all, and sorry to say it, bud, but she's the
one." The rest of my friends agreed. Part of me wanted away from "the one."
The one meant settling down. The one meant commitment. The one meant
complete honesty forever. Part of me wanted to use it all to scare her away
from the insecure and vain young man who sat in front of her. The other part
just wanted to see if she'd stay.

"I was born without a soft spot," I said. That came out easy.

"You've told me that. That's how you got your scars," she said without a
hitch in her voice or a hiccup of thought. We'd been intimate enough within
the first few months of our relationship for her hands to wander through my
hair and for her fingers to touch the cross-hatched pink ridges that either
dented downward into my skin on the top of my head or rose above my skin
on the back of my head from ear to ear.

The first time she touched my scalp, she sat on my lap in her dorm room
that she had rented for her summer internship on the campus of the University
of Utah. Roommates she hadn't known before slept in their beds outside her
closed door. We had gone out earlier, and on our third or fourth date when
we got back to her dorm, while sharing music on her stereo, she sat on my lap
and ran her fingers through my hair. The moment she touched the scar on the
back of my head, I pulled her hands away and warned her that there were more
to come and told her about being born without a soft spot, about the lumps
that made up the landscape of my head and the scarring from the surgery. She
put her hands back into my hair and rubbed her fingers along the scars. We
talked until the morning sunlight came through the windows. We shared everything. Almost everything.

"Well, that's not the whole story," I said.

"What's the whole story?" she asked. The waiter came by and gave us our
sweet-and-sour chicken and fried rice. The smell of fried batter and sweet,
sweet sauce nearly made me cough.

"Well," I stumbled. "When I was eighteen, I was scared of losing all my
hair and stuff."

She took a bite of her chicken, and her face puckered up.

"What?" I said, nervous that she had already known and didn't want to
hear that her assumptions were true.

"This is really bad chicken," she said, as if I were standing in front of a
judge begging for acquittal and the judge was picking his fingernails in disin-
terest.

I took a bite, happy for the extra moment.

"You were eighteen and ... ?" she asked.

"I was eighteen and I got a hair transplant to cover up the scar on the top of my head," I blurted out between a taste of sweet-and-sour. "The scar on the back of my head is from that."

She looked at me from across the table. Her eyes scanned the front of my scalp, and she was quiet.

"I don't care," she said.

I don't know what I wanted from her. The childish boy in me wanted her to run away to leave me to my youth, and the lovesick boy in me wanted her to cry with empathy or something.

"What do you mean, you don't care?" I asked.

"I just don't care, really," she said, and then she topped it off with, "Women are different than men."

"What?" I was confused.

"Women don't care about those kinds of things," she said. "At least smart women."

"Women, or you?" I asked.

"I'm a woman," she said with laughter in her throat.

I was frustrated. Really frustrated. I wanted more. A bigger scene. More to-do about the whole thing. But all I got was "women don't care about those kinds of things."

We ate our gross Chinese food, and I pestered her for more of her inner feelings about what I had told her until we walked back out onto the street that night and wandered up the slick, wet cobbles of the little Irish town. She had finally started to react to the conversation. She was annoyed by my pestering more than anything.

As we walked she grabbed my hand and said, "You could shave tomorrow and look like Frankenstein's monster [the English major in her knew the difference between the doctor and his creation] and I wouldn't care."

"You mean you don't care if I'm attractive?" Her words had brought back the same insecurity that rumbled through my head when I was eighteen—I cared more about being attractive than being me. A beautiful woman walked beside me in the bright Irish moonlight, had confessed her love for me, said she would love me no matter what I looked like, and I was angry.

"So you don't think I'm attractive?" I asked. As if I lived on the edges of her eyelids, I could feel her eyes roll backward in their sockets. It was one of those moments when I knew I was being awful and horribly transparent, but I couldn't keep myself from saying what I was saying.

"'No, Kase. I don't think you're attractive.' Is that what you want me to say?"

"No, but is that the truth?"

"Ugh," she muttered. "You could shave it all off tomorrow and I would still think you were attractive."

This calmed me a bit, comforting my childish insecurity enough to squeeze her hand and walk to the B and B.

"Except women don't care about those kinds of things," she said one last time before we walked through the front door.

The conversation hung in the cold air of autumn in Ireland. I didn't know if I really believed her.

The Ridge

The metopic suture, the thin line of pliable bone and tissue that runs downward from the anterior fontanel through the center of the forehead and stops above the brow line, over the latter half of the twentieth century and beginning of the twenty-first century has moved ahead of unilateral coronal synostosis in number of occurrences, making it the second most common type of synostosis, just behind sagittal synostosis. The early closure, as noted in the medical chapter, pulls all the forehead bone toward the closed suture and creates a triangular shape of the frontal bones, like a book placed spine up to a hold a page. The closure of the metopic suture, in medical terms, is called trigronocephaly—*trigonon*, Greek for "triangle," and *kephale*, Greek for "head," and *metopon*, Greek for "forehead"—was termed by H. Welcker in 1862, and because its accurate description, like that of "plagiocephaly" and "scaphalocephany," the term has stuck.

The metopic suture stands out from the other sutures, however, as a suture that is supposed to close early, usually beginning its closure in the third month of an infant's life and being zipped up with solid bone by the eighth month of child's life, which is why many surgeons doubt the necessity of surgical intervention to release a prematurely closed metopic suture, at least if the trigonocephaly is mild to moderate, noting that the problem may just work itself out or that the closure isn't too far ahead of the curve, so the child shouldn't suffer any physiological, mental, or developmental problems later in life—most agree that the very mild cases of trigonocephaly need not be released, but at what point the trigonocephaly is severe enough to require surgery to avoid physiological or developmental delays is highly debatable and if there is a raging debate in the world of craniosynostosis repair this would be at the heart of it.

The premature closure of the suture does what any set of mountain ranges does: at the point of impact between the once moveable bone plates, the ossification of the bone creates a very visible angle (should be differentiated from a metopic ridge) at the center of the forehead. Since the bone rises up and closes at the center of the forehead, leaving no room for the necessary expansion of the brain beneath the frontal bones, the brain pushes the bones out laterally to compensate for the other bones that are still expanding along the unfused sutures of the skull. In more than half the cases, the anterior fontanel has closed prematurely as well. Many times, again depending on the severity of the closed metopic suture, deficient lateral orbital rims (deficient bones in the eye socket) make the skull around the eyes highly susceptible to both the forward expansion of the skull outward above the eye and the deep indentations of the skull behind the eyes. And in many of the most severe cases, the lateral cantal angles (the angle where the upper and lower eyelids meet) can rise on the skull to abnormally high levels. Basically, with the closure of the metopic suture any and all of the orbital walls and orbital rims are susceptible to hypertolism, retrusion, or indentation, and this is why doctors pay, or should pay, very close attention to any eye issues or seeing issues that arise in the child's young life. Since all of this contributes to less room in which the brain can grow, surgery to release the suture, as with other sutures, must be seriously considered by all parties.

Over the last decade and a half, after looking at 100 patients and comparing them to the general population researchers believe that metopic synostosis happens in about 1 out of 5,200 births. Males, like the larger numbers for all synostosis, outnumber females 2 to 1, and researchers have found that 10 out 179 cases involved a family history of synostosis, but they are hesitant to say that the birth defect is hereditary, as there are so many other reasons why children are born with metopic synostosis, and in one study of more than eight hundred children, researchers found that older mothers and low birth weight elevated the risk of metopic synostosis.

The same question always comes up when it comes to the premature closure of the suture, and most of the time it comes up because mothers and fathers wonder if they did something wrong, if they played a part in the etiological development of their child's craniosynostosis, and, with complete honesty, the answer could be yes, even though it typically isn't yes. Most researchers believe there are three etiological reasons for the early closure of the metopic suture specifically.

First, the most widely recognized theory for the early closure of the metopic suture is that the bone itself carries the "disease" or osseous pathology (the study of disease within the bone) that happens at the beginning of the pregnancy. The cause of the pathology can stem from many different seeds: most believe these seeds are genetic, metabolic, and, yes, pharmaceutical in nature. In metopic synostosis specifically, all of these pathological factors have been present. Studies have shown heredity in a small percentage of children, others have shown thyroid hormone replacement therapy as a cause, while others have shown the use of pharmaceutical drugs during the early development of the fetus that spurs the birth of the disease in the bone. One drug that many researchers have pointed to is valproate, which is used to treat mothers who are prone to seizures or migraine headaches or have psychiatric conditions such as bipolar disorder. The ingestion of folic acid has bleeped on the radar of many researchers as a pathological cause of metopic synostosis, but as of yet there has been no proof of this theory.

Second, one factor that many mothers blame themselves for, but shouldn't, is the limited amount of room in the pelvic region. This theory, having long been believed and supported by the scientific community, places the burden on the constraint of the fetus's head during gestation. Drs. J.M. Smith, Jr., and D.W. Smith in an extensive study in the early eighties found one child was stuck at the bottom of a bicornuate uterus, a heart-shaped uterus, and another child was wedged between his two twins throughout his life in the uterus. Recent studies have confirmed that this pressure in the uterus may correlate with a premature ossification of the metopic suture.

The third element that researchers use to explain metopic synostosis is the malformation of the brain. This theory states that if the frontal lobes of the child are malformed then very little space at the front of the skull would be needed to house the frontal lobes and this would limit the signals to the bone centers and cause the suture to fuse early, the skull believing that it didn't need to keep growing as there was plenty of room for the malformed frontal lobes. There have been studies that show that children with metopic synostosis, even if they had corrective surgery to give the brain enough room to grow, have suffered from developmental delays on the neurodevelopmental spectrum, meaning that the frontal lobes may have been the cause of the problem and that their problematic development happened before the closing of the suture.

All three theories show one thing: there is plenty of proof that the cause of metopic synostosis cannot be pinned down to one seminal problem but to many possible problems during gestation.

Sadly, some researchers believe the highest rate of neurological development delays or problems comes with those children with synostosis who suffer from metopic synostosis, or trigonocephaly. Studies in 1968 and in 1981 reported that developmental delays occurred twice as much in children with metopic synostosis as they did in children with sagittal or coronal synostosis and that nearly 20 percent of children with the population of "trigono-cephalies" reported some kind of neurodevelopmental delays or stunting, and some have stated that the percentage can be as high 61 of those with trigono-cephaly who suffer from neurological delays, while many dispute there is any evidence of this at all. They blame ICP for the neurological delays. Second only to children with multi-suture synostosis, children with metopic synostosis have been, in at least one extensive study, found to have the highest occurrences of increased ICP at 19 percent. That extra pressure on the brain does no good for the children's development. But as noted before when talking about why the metopic suture might close early, doctors still believe that the problems in neurodevelopment might occur before the suture closes. One study found that of those with trigonocephaly who were operated on, 32 percent of those children showed delays. Of those children in the mild range who were not operated on, 23 percent showed delays, backing up the theory that the delays did not come about because of the craniosynostosis but were already present in the brain preossification.

Dr. Fearon, however, believes that the jury is still out on developmental delays associated with craniosynostosis. He is far from saying that there is no correlation and tackles the question with honesty and candor, but he urges parents to look at their decision in a more holistic, rounded way:

> So probably the most likely reason for it is some kind of intruder con-strain and while there are a lot of doctors that believe that kids with craniosyn-ostosis or, and I'm just limiting my remarks to single suture synostoses, but I can get into more complicated if you want. But most are, there's been kind of additional thinking that kids may be more likely to have a development delay or behavioral problems. I just don't believe this to be the case and I follow my patients until the kids are teenagers, so I think I have a pretty good sense of it, but this is being borne out now and some studies that are coming out where if you look at a lot of kids with craniosynostosis, the percentage of kids that have behavioral development problems is significantly different from what you'd see if you just went to any school system and just took all the kids out of third grade and measured them. And I think the jury's still out, but my guess is that if you have it, you just need to have the suture released.
>
> And the two reasons that we operate on kids that have this condition are 1) we can see that the skull takes an abnormal shape with a suture fused shut and it seems it doesn't get better and we now know it probably gets a little bit worse and so 2) is just to normalize appearance so kids will interact with their peers normally, and while that sounds sort of superficial, it's really important, I mean if you have a condition that you look really different than other kids and they're teasing you, you don't want to go to school and it can affect your whole

life. So it's, that's a pretty compelling reason to do it. But the reason I think most parents hand this most prized possession in their life over to a surgeon and say, "I've brought my kid," is because they're worried about the effect it can have on the brain. And there we don't stand on as firm scientific ground.

Early on surgeons focused on pressure, intracranial pressure being an issue, and in the early seventies a couple of studies in Europe were done where every kid and baby that had it, and they'd measure pressure, and surprisingly they found only a small percentage of kids had raised pressure, somewhere between 5 and 15 percent. Now the problem with this study is we don't know what normal pressure is in an infant and we don't know how high it gets or has to get and for how long before it would cause some irreversible damage, but it's one thing we could measure, so we're measuring it. And, and really I don't care if my child has elevated pressure. Really, I mean I'd rather they be normal, but I really want my child to grow up normally. And the thinking is that elevated pressure reduces blood flow to the brain and that reduces the oxygen delivery or the glucose delivery and that affects the function of the brain and, and I mean that's the sequence that we worry about. The problem is the thing we worry the most about, the development, is the thing we are least good at measuring.

I tell a lot of my patients, you know, they say that the old saying that kids in school who gets A's work for kids who got B's and kids who got C's own the company. It's another way of saying that, at least in school, by the way they measure development you're missing some really bright kids that weren't performing well there but are capable of other strengths. We can't measure creative intelligence, artistic intelligence, social intelligence; all these different things we can't measure. So that part of it we're on weaker ground, but newer studies are looking at cerebral blood flow and there are suggestions that regionally under the fused suture there's a reduced blood flow that increases afterwards. So it seems there is some evidence to suggest we're doing the right thing aside from just making people look normal, right?

There's nothing cosmetic about it [surgery], but it raises an interesting point, and that is one of the sutures normally closes in every kid; it's the metopic suture. So if you do a CAT scan on every kid, every ten-month-old, 100 percent of them or close to 100 percent will have a fused metopic suture, so craniosynostosis is a normal process in every kid, but when it occurs early enough that it can impair that growth you get a triangular-shaped forehead and that's what we have to treat; the more the skull shape has evolved the more you have to think that "my child's not going to look normal" or there's going to be an effect on the brain. And the reason it's important is this suture when it closes sometimes can close with a raised ridge, but it still hasn't impaired growth, but when you see this raised ridge people think craniosynostosis and you get an X-ray the suture's fused and you get people that want to operate, and that's just sort of an appearance thing and you don't want to operate for those … [reasons]. I mean you want to operate when the appearance is enough that it's going to affect how your child's going to interact with other kids or if it's going to affect the brain; that's got to be the litmus test of whether you do surgery or not.

But the methods doctors now use to release the suture have become very common and very successful. Most doctors perform a variation of the fronto-supraorbital advancement and remodeling. After the skin is removed and anesthesia is provided, the doctors remove the frontal bone of the skull and then remove the supraorbital bar (the bony ridge or bar above the eye sockets). A wedge is cut out of the posterior midline and the bar is bent into a more horizontal shape to correct the angle of the orbits around the eyes.

"This movement increases the inter-orbital distance, thus eliminating the need for an interpositional bone graft. A unicortical posterior bone graft is subsequently used though to stabilize the midline open wedge osteotomy. A closed wedge osteotomy is performed lateral of the lateral orbital wall, by which an increase of the fronto-temporal angle is achieved. The temporal fragments of the bar are then moved forward in a 'tongue-in-groove' fashion," according to Dr. Jacques van der Meulen. After that, the surgeon cuts the frontal bone down the center, where the metopic suture should have been, and places it in to fit with the newly shaped supraorbital bar. This procedure takes care of many issues. First, it releases the suture so the brain can grow. Second, it reshapes the forehead for aesthetic purposes. And third, it reshapes the orbital walls to ensure that the eyes grow in a way that they naturally should.

There are, of course, many different procedures to release the suture, as a walk into the office of any craniofacial surgeon would show.

The Sound

Hidden behind the curtain, the beeps and lights and surgeons and nurses bopped up and down around her; they pulled Charlie from her belly, her husband Tommy, holding her hand during the procedure.

"That's strange," a nurse said, and shrugged her shoulders in bafflement and confusion.

The first words that Robyn heard from the mouths of the medical professionals who pulled her newborn son from her were, "That's strange. I've never seen that before." I heard the echo of the nurse telling my mom, "Your baby is going to be a retard," when Robyn talked about that day. A small slip from the mouth of a professional can burrow downward into the heart of a mother who had just given birth to a new child, it can wiggle its way through her psyche, and while years will pass and the mom can put it aside, those first words never leave. As if the child were some other type of being, and as if Robyn and her husband weren't standing there, and as if the medical professionals had found out that Google Maps had pointed them in the wrong direction, they said, "That's strange." Two words that no mother wants to hear when her child is first seen. More appropriate word combinations would have been "he's healthy," "he's beautiful," or "say hello" or "congratulations on your new child."

"That's strange" sounds a lot like "it's alive."

The nonchalant shrug of the shoulders left Robyn and Tommy wondering what was so "strange" about their newborn son. Robyn Howard, like many mothers, wanted a natural birth. She wanted her child to come into the world without the use of drugs or tools or a C-section. Charlie's breach changed that, and a week after the doctors saw that little Charlie was lodged in tight, his head pointing upward in the womb, the doctors scheduled a C-section for the next Monday. After the C-section, when the nurse blurted out, "That's strange," she

99

noticed the closing of Charlie's metopic suture. Robyn and Tommy held Charlie in their arms. He was wrapped in a blue and white blanket, and his eyes were bright. He was tiny. And the trigonocephaly was noticeable, his forehead coming together in a triangle shape above his eyes, but the doctors waited one month to make sure that the overhang of the forehead, the prominence of the brow, and the closeness of the eyes weren't present strictly because of the pressure of the breach and would work themselves out. He was diagnosed with craniosynostosis at his one-month checkup, after both Robyn and her pediatrician did research separately and both came into the checkup with the diagnosis.

Many pediatricians don't recognize craniosynostosis when they see it, many of them continue to miss it when the babies come into their offices, and many misdiagnose it. Evidence of this has been found in my own research across this country where pediatricians are educated by the mothers of children with craniosynostosis. Is this a knock on pediatricians? Of course not, but it is a recognition that the resources online have helped a lot of families find the proper diagnosis and treatment for their children.

A mother's guess, right now, is as good as anyone's as to why has suture fused. Robyn believed in her heart that because Charlie was breach in the middle of a perfect pregnancy his position closed his metopic suture and pushed his brow severely down over his brow line, shifting the ridges of his bone and eyes and center of his nose, and at this point in the study of the causes of craniosynostosis, and while there are many reasons why this could have happened, her theory cannot be disproven.

"I'm so thankful for my pediatrician. She didn't know right away, but she recognized that something was wrong and went and found and sent us to specialists. I've heard too many stories about pediatricians just telling parents everything is fine when the moms and dads know something is wrong," Robyn said, a fire flared up in her mind, trying to protect all of those other families who need the right advice and diagnosis.

Seattle Children's Hospital said "moderate to severe metopic." This diagnosis is key to a child born with metopic craniosynostosis, as it is the one synosed suture for which doctors debate the necessity of releasing the bone. In Charlie's case, there was no real option of no surgery, which is always a benefit to two parents who stand in the doctor's office when the doctor says, "We need to operate." Charlie had no real option as the severity of his closure was present at birth and would lead to problems. But those parents who are told that their metopic child is mild to moderate and must make a decision face a whole new level of mind- and heart-tearing decisions, above the most common decision: to operate at all.

"We were so fortunate that we didn't have a choice. I've talked to so many moms who were given the choice and have heard the anguish in their stories over the decision that they had to make," Robyn said.

Robyn had read the horror stories about the what-ifs, the chance of death, the chance of HIV, the chance of complications, but her surgeons at Seattle Children's Hospital were much more gentle and avoided that conversation and trusted that the parents would read the disclosure for the surgery and see it themselves without having to hear again from the doctors, unlike the what-if lady who still appears in Summer Ehmann's nightmares.

Charlie was operated on at nine months. By the time he had been brought into the hospital for surgery, his head had fully developed its trigonocephaly. As if someone had pinched the front of his forehead and held it for the first three months of his life, his head looked like a basketball that had been squeezed into the shape of a traffic cone at one end. That said, Charlie had a smile that could light up a room and bright blue eyes that stopped people in their tracks, but when people are stopped in their tracks they do very little to help.

"No matter how much your family loves you and gives you support, they just don't know what I was actually going through." Others didn't help at all, asking the young parents questions like, "How could you let them do this to your kid?" or saying, "He looks just fine," or, "I don't see any reason to operate," or, "I read that children with a lazy eye like Charlie's can be fixed without surgery," or, the worst of all, "Are you doing this for you or are you doing it for him?"

"People don't know what to say to a mom and dad who have a child who has to go through this," Robyn said. And people come out of the real woodwork to try to dissuade families from surgery. They come in fast and hard and with options that if they really knew about was going on they would never suggest. One natural medicine practitioner said that she could "fix" Charlie by performing massage therapy on the affected suture and release it from its synostosis.

"I'm all for natural medicine and therapy," Robyn said, "but come on; it's bone fused together. There is no way that massaging the scalp is going to release the bone." Robyn and Tommy, Charlie hammering fake nails between them and climbing on anything he could climb on and jump off of, exchanged glances back and forth. Rolls of eyes communicated memories and thoughts and what to say next. Like any couple who had been through hardships together, one began to talk about how "some people still don't get it" and the other gave an example to prove how some people "still don't get it." The anxiety built up by the upcoming surgery, the snippy comments from loved ones, and the naivety of those who had no idea what just might happen to Charlie if he didn't have corrective surgery began to build up like a pile of resentment.

While Robyn and Tommy had no option, as the doctor said Charlie must have surgery, and while they were relieved of nights of asking themselves if the surgery was necessary or if they were making the right decision because of the severity of the closure of the metopic suture, there was always an option to not have the surgery at all, the metopic suture controversy aside. What those people did was plant that little seed of doubt into Robyn's and Tommy's heads. It sits. It takes in nutrients. And it grows. The Howards had months to wait from diagnosis to surgery. Just like a growing season, those seeds had time to sprout, to stretch their healthy vines into the solid decision of the Howards and do their best to break apart the cement-like solidarity of the Howards' decision. Those rapturous vines, just weeks before surgery, manifested themselves as body tics, insomnia, stomach cramping, and migraines for Robyn, and, unless parents have had a sick child or a child who has needed life-altering surgery during infancy they can never really understand, and as I type this I know that I could never understand. Those feelings, very understandably, take different forms throughout nine months of fermenting worry.

"It was hard, I mean we almost got mad at people who had these perfect children and had the perfect first few months of parenthood. Even though that wasn't really fair to them, we couldn't help but resent them a bit. It all seemed unfair," said Tommy.

At a mothers' group, surrounded by moms and their children, all about the same age as Charlie, Robyn sat in the room and listened to the worries and complaints of all the mothers: they worried about earaches and colds and diaper rash and all the little worries that come with parenthood. Robyn, probably one of the genuinely sweetest people I have met in this long journey across the country, got angry at those mothers. She saw the worry on their faces, shown in the downturned lips and scrunched brows, and thought, *I remember just wanting to smack some of them. They were complaining about things that to them were a big deal, but I couldn't stop myself from thinking that you don't have to worry about your child having to have major head surgery.*

A natural researcher, Robyn bought every book on the market that talked about the first few months of raising a child. She stood in the aisles of bookstores and thumbed through copies of *What to Expect the First Year* and others in the same vein that make the rows of books on the bookshelves resemble a rainbow of knowledge produced by doctor after doctor and psychologist after psychologist, but none of the books, as her finger ran down the table of contents, as she flipped to the chapters about "complications" during the first year, and as she read subheading after subheading of complications, said anything about cranial complications or "missing soft spots" or closed sutures. Her response was only anger and surprise. Every pediatrician runs his or her fingers over a child's head. It is common practice to place fingers on the fontanels and search for soft tissue, so why wouldn't there be a common subheading within all of these books that at least mentioned that there was a possibility that there might be no "soft spots" and that this was the result of a major birth defect that can affect the child physically, mentally, and, at the very least, psychosocially?

This completely baffled me. So I picked up five or six of the most popular baby books and began my search for any mention of soft spots or sutures or the importance of the pediatrician's examination when it came to the cranial sutures throughout the first year of the newborn's life. *The Experts' Guide to the Baby Years*, a well-written and fun book overall, stamped with "EXPERT" in bright red letters on the front, had chapters about writing a will, helping an older child meet a new sibling, and how to maintain your sex life, subjects that are very important with a newborn, as I know, having just brought one home two years ago, but don't help in the overall developmental growth of the child or warn parents about the dangers of a critical birth defect that touches 1 in 1,700 children. The book has very nice but short chapters about choosing a pediatrician, choosing the right car seat, and breast-feeding. Then there are very well-written and important chapters that cover keeping the baby healthy, looking for signs of illness, recognizing and treating colic, and, very important, a three-page chapter about reducing the risk of SIDS. Having known families who have lost their children to SIDS, I realize this chapter cannot be undervalued, nor is it my intent to devalue the author's emphasis on SIDS or any other illness—my heart cries out to any family who has suffered the loss of a child to SIDS. But it is in this chapter where the authors circle around the importance of skull development when they discuss the need to adjust the angle of the bed and limit the time in carriers to avoid misshaping the head—positional plagiocephaly—since the child will need to sleep on her back to avoid the SIDS. A mention of skull development would only enhance the chapter and the parents' knowledge of why we are now placing children on their backs to sleep. The expert does an awesome job with this four-page chapter, but most of the book is spent delving into how to be a stylish mom, how to wear your baby, and how to do yoga with your baby. The index said nothing of fontanels or soft spots or sutures, even though craniosynostosis occurs in less than 1 in 1,700—I'm guessing, across the nation, a number bigger than those who need advice on how to search for a full-time, live-in nanny (another chapter in the book).

The Happiest Baby on the Block, a much less hipster-style book than *The Experts' Guide to the Baby Years,* is much more straightforward and informative and has a very nice section on SIDS, but this book does not mention plagiocephaly and does not talk in any way about looking for signs of craniosynostosis.

These books do their jobs. They inform the largest audience about the most common problems, misconceptions, and worries; however, what is a mom to do when she looks down at her newborn child, her pediatrician has cleared the baby of any problems, but the mother knows that something is wrong with the child's head? The books say nothing, not even a mention of closed "soft spots" or sutures, when all they would need to do was say something brief but pointed like, "If your child's skull shape looks different from other baby's skull shapes, or your family's skull shape, ask your pediatrician about plagiocephaly or craniosynostosis. Chances are, there is absolutely nothing wrong, but it never hurts to ask at your next checkup." Simple wording like this at the end of a chapter that talks about illnesses would do three things: it would give parents of children with craniosynostosis something to grasp on to to ease their worries, it would alert parents to complications of the skull, and if worded in this tone, without creating a rush of unnecessary paranoia, it would keep parents, like Robyn, from using Google as their first reference, as the Internet, typically on the first search, flashes the most extreme and most complicated cases of craniosynostosis, as well as tons of misinformation, when most children with craniosynostosis are on the less extreme side of the spectrum. Robyn fumed about these books, fumed about the lack of solid information out there, and steamed about some pediatricians who don't actually look for the birth defect.

Charlie had a full CVR. The fear of the surgery for months was always there. It lingered in Charlie's parents' minds when they were at the mothers' group, while Tommy was at work, and even after the surgery had come and gone.

Charlie's pre-surgery scans were smooth, with all clean, clear sagittal, coronal, and lambdoid sutures and shields of smooth bone surround them like they had been polished by the hand of a talented crystal maker, but as if the sculptor had forgotten the metopic suture, the bone is clean and smooth and in one unbroken piece of bone above Charlie's brow. His post-scan looked much, much different. They took bone from the back of his head and created a new brow line for little Charlie. They reconstructed his eye sockets by bringing them outward and farther apart. Then they reshaped his entire head to match that which is considered normal. The result of all this surgical handiwork left a scan without the smoothness of the pre-scan photo, with ridges and holes and cuts on the front half of his skull above his brow line. Like two ships that ride on a rough sea, the cuts in the bones look like waves cutting into the bows of the ships, and above them two flag-like shapes, like those hoisted from the ships into the sky, extend backward into the once smooth sea of bone. Below the ships of rattled bone, as if the doctors took two ball-shaped pieces of Play-Doh and rolled them in their hands until they became long and narrow like noodles and placed them, one on top of the other, they created a more prominent brow line. Below the new brow line, more cracks and cuts and pieces reshaped the little boy's head and let the skull grow.

During surgery, Tommy took a quick bathroom break while he and Robyn waited for their son, who lay in the operating room. There, in the bathroom, Tommy washed his hands, looked down at the water and watched it fall between his fingers and the soap turn white on his palms. Something in the mixing of soap and water and the coolness of the liquid that ran over his fingers brought everything home, made the moment real, and broke him down. That's when he lost it, when he truly recognized what was happening just a few walls away. The world in which he was living, one in which his son currently lived without the top part of his skull, came crashing down on Tommy and he wept. He stood in the bathroom and let it out for four or five minutes, his tears mixing with the soapy water, but then he looked at himself in the mirror and pulled in the outward symptoms of emotion and pain and worry before he returned to Robyn in the waiting room to hold her tight and be strong until the boy returned.

As Charlie hammered with his toy hammer beside me in the Howards' front room, the questions suddenly turned to me and Charlie's dad had one specific question that I could see he had been wanting to ask.

"Do you have younger siblings? I'm curious," he asked. Charlie pounded wooden pegs into his wooden workbench. He smiled and hammered and giggled and hammered. I knew they wanted me to say yes, to say that after I was born my parents went ahead and had a third child, but I couldn't. My older brother nearly killed my mom during his birth, and after I had recovered from my craniosynostosis and my month-long stays in the hospital to clear my lungs, my parents made the easy decision for my dad to get a vasectomy. Tommy's and Robyn's eyes watched me for a moment.

"No, no more after me," I said. Their eyes dropped a bit.

"It is all still present for us because we worry about having a second child, and we want to," Tommy said. "It's still there because we have a deep fear about a second kid."

Charlie hammered away beside me. The sound echoed through the room, and all it took to find levity in the moment was a glance at the little boy, happy and healthy, hammering away in the living room, but his mom and dad laid it out clearly that they didn't know if they were brave enough to go through all of it again. From what I had seen, in family after family, they didn't have children after they had a child with craniosynostosis. If they had two children and the second child had craniosynostosis, they had no more. If they had seven children and the seventh child was born with craniosynostosis, they did not have an eighth child, and if their first had craniosynostosis that needed to be corrected, a second child was very rare.

Throughout my conversation with the Howards, it continually swung back toward Robyn's worries for other parents. She worried about those who didn't have a world-class children's hospital, about how they had to be overwhelmed with stress and with travel and with recovery. There, again, was that fire that flared up in a woman who if I met on the street would seem like one of the gentle ones, and I'm sure she is, but when she thought about misdiagnosed children or undiagnosed children her motherly guard came up, and came up fast. She worried about those who have surgeons who rarely perform the surgery and whose children have to have more than one surgery and travel to a more practiced doctor after the first doctor didn't do the surgery well. She worries about them all, and her voice rises.

"I can't imagine your mom being alone, without the support that is out there today," Robyn said. She looked at me. And her eyes saddened, not for me but for my mom. "I just can't imagine not having anyone else to talk to about this who had gone through the same thing. I don't think my worry about his head will go away. Every time I touch him, I think of it. It has to be the same for your mom."

Charlie was swollen after surgery. He was black-and-blue. It wasn't just the flesh and bone around his eyes that swelled up, but Robyn explained that his actual eyes swelled outward too. His scar was fresh and bright and covered in stitches, and the swelling and black-and-blue, unlike those of many other children, stuck around for many weeks. Tommy got looks from others at the store weeks after the surgery. People looked at him as if he had struck his child, Charlie's eyes swollen and a hat covering his scar. One lady at the zoo asked if Charlie had fallen. She looked down at the zigzagged scar that ran from one ear, over the top of the head, and then down to the other ear and asked if the scar came from the random fall of a boy who just had begun to walk.

The Howards stayed in the PICU alone for one night after Charlie's surgery and then were moved into a room that was made for two young patients. Each night they had new roommates, and each night they had to listen to the cries of other parents and other infants. One night, a baby with spina bifida lay in a bed next to them. Another night, a child with cancer. The Howards just wanted to go home. Exhaustion had finally taken them. Charlie lay in his bed with his head covered up. He had tubes connected to him. And they would be released the Friday after a Tuesday morning surgery. Charlie's life would start again in a short couple weeks, but the Howards didn't just want to go home to get their son into his own bed and start that new, bright phase of their life with their son whose brain could not grow in the way it was supposed to. They wanted to go home because their hearts had wept for all the other children in the PICU.

Earlier that year, Robyn had gotten so frustrated with the moms who whined about teething and boogers and sleepless nights. They frustrated her with their tiny worries. But as the Howards walked out of the PICU that Friday afternoon, Charlie snuggled beneath his father's arm and swelled up, Robyn and Tommy felt relief and sorrow, a mix of emotions available to parents whose child had just had major cranial surgery and who knew that every child in the PICU had it worse and might never leave the hospital or live a normal life.

"It was hard being there so long. It was hard to be on that floor and knowing that ours was not as bad. I mean, he just had major surgery, but when we saw what others were going through, it was very humbling. Nothing prepared us for that," she said.

* * *

That night, I drove down I-5 and back to a house Mary and I rented on the round beaches of the Puget Sound. We had been visiting from Kansas. Since we had recently moved from Tacoma to Kansas, we stayed a week to visit friends and for me to get some interviews done. My mom and dad flew up and stayed with us in the rental house. This interview, just like the rest of the interviews, took a toll on me, twisting my heart with the struggles of parents and their children and their complications. When I pulled into the driveway, I was mentally and emotionally tired. I sat and waited before I went in, trying to pull myself away from the interview with the Howards. And I thought I had. Until the five of us sat down to dinner in a mom-and-pop Italian restaurant in Tacoma and had a couple glasses of red wine to relax after a long day of interviews and reliving months of stress and worry with families during interviews and I began to tell my parents about the interview. The wine loosened the tears from my mom's eyes.

The East River

The Queensboro Bridge stretched out toward Queens, reaching across the East River and leaning into the another skyline of buildings, and I sat alone and thought about the young family the Hewitts, whom I had just had coffee with in a café across the street from NYU Medical Center and about my little family who roamed the rooms of the Children's Museum uptown. Seagulls and pigeons bounced on the posts of the pier. It was early January. Runners with legs covered in tights and heads covered in hats ran along the brick of the waterfront. People lined up to catch the ferry. It wiggled across the river from the opposite pier. Families got on, and it wiggled back again. Four benches sat on the deck, spaced twenty feet from each other, and each was occupied by one person. I sat on my bench holding my briefcase close to me for warmth. An older man sat on the bench closest to me, about twenty feet away, and fed the pigeons, and a young women sat on the bench past him. She leaned back, brushed her hair from her forehead, and let the sunlight fall onto her skin. Although it was cold, it was one of those mornings that if you gave the sun enough time on your face it would warm your skin. To my left, another man sat alone, and pulling out a sandwich from his jacket, he glanced over at me, catching my eyes on him. He shrugged and fed half the bread to the surrounding birds that walked up and down the promenade.

The world slowed for an hour. The water lay calm in front of me, the city rattled with honks, and the wind whispered between the buildings behind me. Clouds dusted the sky above the buildings in Queens across the river. And I thought about that family again. And my little family again. The world slowed down for an hour even though I sat at the edge of one of the busiest cities in the world. I had to wait to meet Dr. Staffenberg, one of the leading craniofacial surgeons in the country, in his office, a meeting that brought on the nerves in my stomach that since I was a child felt like someone grabbed ahold of my intestines and twisted and twisted and twisted, but that morning on the pier with the water out in front of me I was able to calm myself. It may have been that I'd used up all my nervousness while waiting out front of NYU Medical for the Hewitts or that while I had tried to build up some kind of wall or immunity to families I talked with, every time I sat down with one and they took me through their journey it drained me, emotionally and physically, so I sat on the east bench and watched New Yorkers walk by on their way to the ferry or sit comfortably on benches and feed the birds.

The time came when I had to stand up and leave the river behind me for another hour or so. I tried to stay in the sunlight as I walked along Third and 23rd—the cold wind that slid along the edges of buildings cut through my clothes when I stepped into the shade. One last time—for just a moment—I looked back at the East River and the buildings on the other side and tried to bring that peace I had there along with me, but it was gone; the nerves had taken ahold of me.

* * *

A little more than two hours earlier, I had hailed a cab from the entrance of our hotel in Times Square, nervous that I would jump on the wrong subway car and end up on the other side of the city, and listened to the taxi driver talk on his cell phone while we headed east toward NYU Medical. I stood at the north entrance of the medical center by the portable toilets and waited for the Hewitts to arrive. Jamie and I had gone back and forth via e-mail for a couple months in order to line up a time and place to meet. Then, as communication in society has evolved, we switched from e-mail to texting as the day got closer. A text let me know that they were finding a parking spot. Jamie and her husband, Stephen, had driven from upstate New York to meet with me, bringing along Jamie's parents to help with the Hewitts' boy, Lucas, while we talked.

A few minutes later, the five of them rounded the corner, the steam of the city rising up from behind them and cars whizzing by behind them. Lucas rode in his stroller pushed by Grandpa, an older man with hair that dropped down out of his ponytail to the middle of his back, and Grandma walked beside them. We all shook hands, everyone a little skeptical of me at first, except for Jamie, their brows furrowing as they examined a man whom they had never met before but who had asked for them to open up their lives and display them on the table of a café, a display of pictures and emotions and scars, emotional and physical.

"I'm John," Lucas's grandpa said, extending his hand outward to me, shaking it, and then pointing to the portable toilets behind us, "and I got to use the john." He laughed at his joke while his wife rolled her eyes, but the simple expression of humor and laughter broke the tension.

"There's a café right there. Would that work?" Jamie asked. I had no better suggestions, so after John got out of the john we headed down the side-walk. We talked about their drive, that I lived in a town in Kansas called Man-hattan, and how my son was also named Lukas. Once we were in the café, the waitress looked at the six of us. She glanced down at two-year-old Lucas, a glance I had seen hundreds of times given to us by hosts and hostesses that said, *I'll find a place for you as far away from other customers as possible.* Two-year-old boys seem to evoke this reaction in restaurants. She sat us at the back of the café by the restroom and kitchen. Jamie and Stephen sat together on one side of the booth and placed Lucas between them in a booster seat, a tac-tical move to keep him between the both of them, another experience that I had become familiar with. Grandma and Grandpa settled in across from them, and I sat in a seat at the end of the table. They stared at me, and to get things started Jamie pulled a stack of photos from her purse and laid them out in front of me. Lucas's grandma shuffled in her seat. Her discomfort spread out across her face when the pictures of Lucas were laid on the table.

The server filled our mugs with cheap, corner-café–style coffee and caught a glimpse of Lucas's CT scans and post-op photos on the table. His head was covered with zigzagged scars. His eyes were swollen nearly shut, and black-and-blue surrounded the fleshy areas that weren't laced in pink and bright red. The server paused for a moment. She couldn't help but squint and purse her lips. She stared for a long couple of seconds before snapping herself out of her stare and asking us if we would like anything to eat. The Hewitts and Lucas's grandparents ordered their meals while I stared down at the photos and sipped my coffee. This moment, when Lucas's head lay out in front of me—when all parents opened up their bags or folders and dropped traumatic photos out in front of me—was not easy. I, like the waitress and even though I have seen thousands of these photos, had to steady myself, look at the photos with a strong heart, and move on to ask questions about the young boy. The best part about the interviews is looking down at the misshapen and recon-structed heads on the table and looking up to see children bouncing around on their parents' laps, writhing with a two-year-old's discontent at not getting what he or she wants, and banging utensils against plates like any other little person would do at a café in New York City when everyone around him wants to talk about serious stuff and all he wants to do is play—that's what I looked up to find Lucas doing, giving his parents the business, and that's what gives me enough joy to move and talk about it all with parents.

The server left with their orders, and the family of five turned back to me. Jamie, as most mothers do, took the lead, shuffling through photo after photo of her son's CT scans, pre-op photos, and post-op photos. She dove into the first few days when they first noticed his misshapen head, she talked about the horror of his diagnosis, and she told me that once the doctors got into surgery they found a much worse scenario than they had expected to find.

Lucas had a rough start; his blood sugar kept dropping, so he had to be taken to the nursery for close observation a couple of times after he was born. During his second trip to the nursery, the doctors and nurses did another examination of Lucas's head and found that the boy "had no soft spots," and this is how they explained it to Jamie and Steve, who waited in their hospital room for the medical staff to bring their son back to them. "No soft spots," was the same thing the doctors told my mom nearly forty years earlier, and while the medical technology has matured and surgical procedures have matured, it seems that communication between doctors and patients still lags way behind, as the parents at the coffee shop that morning could have just as easily digested and understood, and probably would have preferred to hear, that one of Lucas's sutures had closed prematurely.

Lucas was born at 1:40 p.m. and was taken away from his mom and dad. He was taken and returned to his parents intermittently for the next nine hours. Luckily, the nurse on staff had a brother who was born with craniosynostosis thirty-five years earlier, and here lies the conundrum that surrounds this birth defect: when a child is born with craniosynostosis, there always seems to be someone who knows someone else who has had it, but if I were to ask twenty people on the street if they knew about the birth defect that occurs in 1 in every 1,700 births in the United States, meaning that there are hundreds of thousands of us out there roaming the streets across the country, very few would actually know that the premature closing of the "soft spots" is even a possibility and therefore they would have no inclination to look for it at birth, as many doctors fail to look for it also. Lucas's forehead was molded into a triangle from the closing of, at least, his metopic suture.

In the hospital right after his birth, he wore a soft green cap that wrapped itself around his head, hiding, at times, during those first few hours, the bulge that pushed outward from his forehead and shadowed his eyes. The skin on the sides of his forehead was pulled tight toward the edge of the triangle at the front of his head. To Jamie and Steve, he was beautiful. To the naked eye, his prominent trigonocephaly was very evident. When it comes to metopic babies and surgery, it is the one suture that has what most would call a "gray" area, as noted by all the specialists I talked to during my research, as the

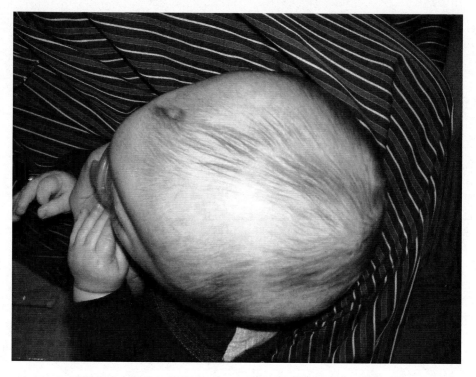

Picture of Lucas pre–surgery for metopic synostosis (courtesy of Jamie Hewitt).

metopic suture closes first and early, mostly closing as early as the first year of life, and many children just need to be watched to make sure there is no ICP or other issues with the early closing of the suture, but there seems to be a large consensus that if a child comes out of the womb with a closed metopic suture the gray area disappears and becomes black and white: a surgery needs to happen to release the suture. Many professionals use the six-month time line. If the triangle appears before six months, chances are the child will need the suture released; if a metopic ridge pops up after six months, the child may need surgery, but the first reaction by medical professionals is to watch the development of the suture and growth of the skull carefully. That said, as all research I came across notes, that "gray" area to operate on children with a metopic ridge, distinguishing between just a ridge and metopic craniosynostosis, is still highly debatable, and the "gray" area does not seem to be shrinking among the medical field. Lucas was not in that gray area. His head pulled and tucked and squeezed and grew outward and backward to account for the strength and rigidity of his stubborn metopic suture that decided to close up while he tossed and turned inside Jamie for nine months.

Thankfully for the Hewitts, and for many others who had children who were born with the birth defect, this nurse had a brother who had surgery thirty-five years earlier and had lived a productive, close-to-normal life. The nurse sat with the young family as Lucas began his life and she told them about her brother, she let them into his life, and she made them feel at ease for at least those first few moments when they found out about their son's birth defect, giving them enough time and information to help them through the first night. She told them that her brother was successful, that he was obnoxious, like any other brother, and that he had a nice family. This was enough for them, as they did their best to fall asleep that night, to at least say, "This is not how we planned it. This is not the popping of champagne, taking of photos, or snuggling all night with our baby like we thought it would be, but it's going to be okay."

That moment of reassurance, while extremely valuable and something that could not be underestimated, was very fleeting. The next day would come and with it more cliffs of fear that the family could not have imagined.

It was an unusually warm day in Rhinebeck, New York, when Lucas was born, topping out at fifty degrees Fahrenheit when that part of the state averages the high thirties that time of year, and it was even warmer the day the ambulance driver told Jamie and Steve that they should go home and shower before heading to Albany, an hour north of Northern Dutchess Hospital, to rejoin Lucas in the NICU at Albany Medical Center. The doctors just couldn't get his sugars to stabilize, coincidentally, like many of the other babies born with premature ossification of their cranial sutures.

"Go home and shower," the ambulance driver said. "You won't be able to see him for a couple hours anyway." Then they took Lucas away, carried him to the ambulance, shut the doors behind them, and left for the capital city.

"So, you're telling me I won't be able to see my child for at least four hours and you're going to take him away from us until then?" Steve asked the doctors and ambulance driver.

"Yes," they told him. "Go home for a while."

They wouldn't let Jamie or Steve ride with Lucas to Albany in the ambulance, so they had to do what the doctor said: they had to say good-bye to their little guy for a while and live their lives without him as he lay in the back of an ambulance and traveled the miles to Albany on his second day of life on November 29, 2010. It was another very warm day for the area, topping out at sixty-three degrees Fahrenheit, the sun peering through the car windows when Jamie and Steve drove home to take a quick shower, as instructed by the ambulance driver to avoid sitting at Albany Medical Center and not being able to see their baby for hours. It takes that long to admit children into the NICU, so Jamie and Steve followed the rules, even though she wanted nothing to do with the separation that was forced upon her and would have given up 100 showers to be in the ambulance with her newly born son.

"This was not how I imagined leaving the hospital: without my baby. That added another blow to what I dreamed it would all be like," Jamie said. Her eyes fell downward to her two-year-old son, who rearranged spoons and forks and knives on the table in the diner. Her hand touched his back, and then, without thought or hesitation, she ran her hand along the top of his head. Steve caressed the two-year-old's back, and Grandma and Grandpa just stared at their daughter and her young family with a gaze of remembrance, calling back those days from a couple years before.

They had crossed the Hudson over the Kingston-Rhinecliff Bridge. Its tall beams arched beneath them, dropping shadows across the water, the sun pushing its rays around the beams' edges on the unusually warm day. The Hudson flowed beneath them around the giant concrete footings that held the bridge high in the air above the river to connect the tree-covered east side of the river to the tree-covered west side of the river.

Outside their apartment, cars lined the street. The sun stayed high in the sky with no clouds to cover it up, and all four of Lucas's grandparents waited for Jamie and Steve to caravan up to Albany.

"We have amazing families," Steve says as he lifts his cup of coffee to his mouth, avoiding the eyes of his in-laws who sit across from him, as compliments to in-laws are always hard to give in person without blushing or starting a chain of compliments back and forth.

The caravan set out first along the New York State Thruway (Highway 87) north toward the state capital. The road paralleled the Hudson River for about twenty miles, weaving past Mount Marion and the Indian Ridge Campsites and Canoe Lake and the maples and pines and oaks that lined the four-lane highway up the interior of the state. The bright oranges and reds and greens of the changing fall trees had begun to fade into gray, and their leaves had begun to depart for the winter, leaving bare branches and lonely limbs to wave at the caravan of cars heading north. They stopped at toll booths and rest stops for food and to use the restroom, none of them in any of the cars aware of what they had passed along the way to see their child or their child's child.

They arrived at Albany Medical Center. Its tall white pillars held the round overhang that welcomed its patients and visitors. Old red brick folded from one edge of the building and merged with plain white and flat walls of the other edge of the building, remnants of generations of add-ons and additions, physical symbols of a hospital that has grown over time, dating back to its days as a medical college in the late 1800s. The caravan came to a halt outside the hospital doors, and though they had headed home, taken showers, and grabbed sandwiches from a rest stop along the way, not even considering staying at home long enough to make food or actually stopping for food along the way, they still had to wait a couple hours for admittance into the NICU to find their boy.

"The NICU is hard," Jamie said. "Compared to the other babies there, Lucas looked good, but it was still torturous to see him there under the lights and not coming home with us that day." Instead of Lucas being wrapped up in a blanket at home, being held in his mother's arms, and living the life his parents had dreamed about, the whole family was instead wrapped up in a world of worry and uncertainty.

At the café in Manhattan, taxis speeding by and ferries honking on the East River outside, Jamie told the story, for the most part, but as she spoke Steve nodded and added little details to their story line, helping her to fill in holes in her memory when she turned his way and asked for help with just her eyes. This type of correspondence and weaving through stories is very common when families retell their stories—husbands typically sit back as the wives talk and then jump in when asked or when a rich memory pops into their minds that they need to share—and I expected that from Jamie and Steve. But more was happening at that table than the common interaction between husband and wife.

Jamie's mom and stepdad tried to play it cool. They did their best to sip their coffee and help out with Lucas by walking around and fiddling around with their eggs and pancakes as if they were having any normal breakfast at any normal café and having any normal conversation, but they were unsuccessful in their efforts. As Jamie and Steve recounted their story, Jamie's mom sighed, moaned, and at one time began to tear up a bit—even though she tried to disguise her wiping away of her tear as an attempt to clean something out of her eye. Jamie's stepdad squinted and frowned and grimaced during certain parts of the story and even added at one point, "Yeah, they told them they should go home and shower, like that would be easy enough for them to do." Like the caravan of cars full of grandparents (Jamie's and Steve's parents) traveled along Thruway 87 toward Albany, following Steve and Jamie's lead, their hearts followed along too, unable to get off the emotional highway that their children navigated that warm day in November.

It was in the NICU that the neurosurgeon took X-rays of Lucas's head to make sure that his sutures had actually ossified and that the shape of his head wasn't developed because of severe case of positional plagiocephely from irregular positioning in the womb. In the neurosurgeon's opinion, the X-rays confirmed craniosyonostosis.

They released Lucas two days later on December 1, 2010, and while the ambulance and the caravan had sunny skies to guide them along the thruway two days earlier, the December sky decided to dump heavy rain on them when they left Albany Medical. They sky was thick with dark clouds, Steve gripped the wheel, his young son riding in the backseat, and rain poured all the way back to their home. The road disappeared in front of them like the rain had washed it away, but Steve white-knuckled his way along the thruway until the family pulled into their driveway to begin the next five months of their lives, which, as for every parent who has had to wait for their child's surgery, would prove the most difficult months of their lives, much more difficult than the first few days of Lucas's life, more difficult than the separation on the road to Albany, and much more difficult than anything the sky could throw at them.

The Hewitts were sent home with instructions that could be translated to, "Don't let your son develop normally until his surgery." They were told to not let him do the things that he would naturally want to do, to ensure that he wouldn't try to do them again after his surgery, when his skull would be fragile. So if they saw him begin to try to roll over or push himself up or do anything that involved mobility, they were told to pick him up, to prevent him from moving around too much, and to, basically, prohibit his body from learning how to develop large motor skills.

"'Just try to keep him a baby as long as you can. Try not to let him develop,'" Steve mimicked the instructions, and chuckled a little bit, one of those chuckles that release frustration.

The worst five months of their lives were upon them. The stress, the worry, and the anticipation took their toll, like they always do, on the mother, her anxiety needing a prescription to settle it down.

"They were horrible," Jamie's mom says of her daughter's worries, "The worst." At the time, the Hewitts felt like they were trying to enjoy every moment with Lucas, because even though odds were low and the doctors were very optimistic, there was a chance that they could lose him during surgery, a warning that the surgeons have to give and gave to the young family. But looking back, Jamie and Steve see the memories and days of those five months completely differently.

"We were robbed of those months," Jamie said. Because of Lucas's condition, they could never truly enjoy those days, the looming cranial surgery bounding across the conscious and, even when they tried to put it out of their mind, their subconscious.

"We never truly got to enjoy him," she said.

While Jamie swam in the worry and fear, Steve did everything he could to not think about it, purposefully trying to stash the worry in the back of his mind, to get it away from his thoughts, all while supporting his wife and loving his child in a way that he felt bonded him and his boy unconditionally and deeper than most other fathers and sons.

"By the time it got to the surgery day, that was easy," Steve said.

Although time dug its heels into the ground and did its best to stall its passing, digging and digging into the sands to prolong the stress of waiting for their child to go under the knife, the Hewitts' dreams and anticipation had become only a stirring of the past: surgery day had come. It was the day they had been waiting for, and it marked the start of another life for them and their son, with a new type of worrying to come their way in the days to come post-op and the months ahead when they would do their best to try to keep their son from damaging his head.

It was early in the morning when Jamie and Steve walked through the front doors of Albany Medical and thirty or more family and friends, including all the grandparents, trickled in behind them with hands full of coffee and snacks and full of support and smiles and kindness. The streets of Albany were filled with people going about their days as they typically go about their days: cars moved and braked in traffic, people walked along the sidewalks in search of the door that would lead them into their day-to-day routine of spreadsheets or meetings or gossip, parents hustled their children to day care or school, as the world around the hospital went about its day as usual, all without a thought of what happened in the hospital down the road. But inside Albany Medical, nurses and doctors roaming the hallways, there was the air of fearful anticipation of starting another chapter in the life of a young boy. On every side of Jamie and Steve, grandmas and grandpas and aunts and uncles and friends flanked them like wingmen following the lead plane into a sea of an unknown battle, hands placed on shoulders and prayers whispered in corners in the waiting room.

Then Lucas was taken away, leaving his mother's arms empty, only to be touched by the outstretched arms of family. There would be pacing and nail biting and jokes to ease the tension. There would be coffee drinking and donut eating and upset stomachs. There would be glance after glance toward the doors that led to the operating room, and for two and a half hours hospital staff would walk through those doors without any news for the crowd that had formed in the waiting room

Just under three hours after they had taken Lucas away, a nurse came to talk with the family.

More than thirty people stood up. Their hearts raced. They were ready to hear what had happened in the OR. Adrenaline pushed through their veins, shocking their systems with that rush of energy and excitement, the feeling of relief only experienced when someone realizes that they have made it through a few of the worst hours, days, and months of their lives.

"We haven't gotten started yet," the nurse said, his voice strong at first but taken over by an apologetic tone by the time he finished telling them that the doctors had yet to begin. Another surgery had gotten started late and had taken longer than they had anticipated, and when that was through, in the pre-op room, under the fluorescent hospital lights, on the white-sheet-covered bed, and beneath a gown made just for babies, Lucas's veins hid from the nurses and anesthesiologist.

"We couldn't find a nerve for the IV," the nurse said, "but we finally found one, and we are taking him in now." The nurse walked back through the double doors and into the operating room, leaving behind him a trail of busted bubbles and the numbness and tingling left in the body after a rush of adrenaline had done its work.

"Oh my gosh, oh my gosh, oh my gosh, we have to do this all over again," Jamie's mom said. A Sisyphean feeling fell over the crowd of people in the waiting room, especially those closest to Lucas and his parents. The wait would begin again, the hours would dig in their heels, and the world outside would go about its day until the neurosurgeon came through the doors and was rushed by waves of Lucas's large family the second he made it into the waiting room.

When the doctors cut into Lucas' head, the zigzag incision and pulling back and forth of the skin, the open head revealed that not only had Lucas's metopic suture closed, but by the time he waited for surgery and was put under the knife other sutures had closed as well. The situation was more complex than the doctors had previously thought, but Lucas was scheduled for a full CVR, so the doctors were prepared to perform the full CVR no matter what. They took off the top of Lucas's head from the brow upward, like carefully taking the lid off an oval glass serving dish, knowing that it is the only lid that would fit the dish and knowing that it had to be handled with the utmost care. They broke the skull apart with a tiny medical hammer. They chipped and designed, crafted and molded, and then put his skull back together on this head. Edges and corners, both round and sharp, reshaped his skull. Like flat rocks pasted onto that same serving dish lid, they put it all back together and closed the very little boy up.

Typically, the doctor takes the parents into a smaller room, sits them down, and tells them how everything went. That day, however, Jamie ran up to him in a full sprint and met him before he could escort her and Steve away. Her supporters all stood up at once like a crowd giving an actor a standing ovation and formed a wall behind her, rows of heads bobbing over and around other heads to hear what the doctor had to say.

"How is he?" Jamie said. She stood within inches of the neurosurgeon, her anticipation and the pride of loved ones behind her overwhelming him.

"Well, I'm not supposed to do it this way," he said. He became flustered.

"How is he?" someone else from the crowd asked.

The doctor, looking at everyone in front of him, pulled away from protocol and answered, "He's doing good. Everything went well."

With these words, Jamie threw her arms around the doctor's neck and thanked him. His face revealed shock and happiness, all wrapped into brows

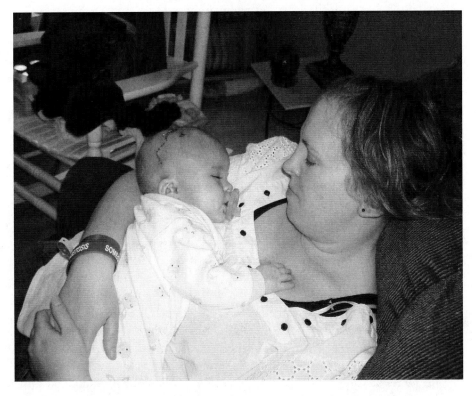

Picture of Lucas post–surgery for metopic synostosis , with mother Jamie Hewitt (courtesy of Jamie Hewitt).

that showed an overall feeling of being completely overwhelmed by the reception he received from Jamie and the crowd behind her. Hugs and kisses and pats on the back swam around the room between family and friends. Right then, right there, the world began to spin again for the Hewitts, and even though Lucas would rip off his bandages in the days following surgery and even though he would be a handful at breakfast that morning in Manhattan, he had bigger handfuls of family to hold him, to stand behind his mom and dad, take him for a walk on the New York streets to placate the busied body of a two-year-old and bring him back just in time for the grown-ups to tear up over eggs and coffee.

The cliché states that it takes a village to raise a child, and this is true, but it is even truer that it takes a village to make it through the traumatic months before and after surgery for craniosynostosis (and other serious, sometimes much more serious, pathologies), and as I have seen over and over again while talking with family after family, it is much more the norm than the exception that while the world goes about its business without even an inkling of what is happening behind hospital doors, people love these little children, and the amount of support that follows them can never be hidden or overstated. The Hewitts and their families and friends are only a small microcosm of the support for families I've seen along this path.

On August 4, 2013, nearly two and half years after Lucas blessed this world, he welcomed his baby brother to the family. Jamie and Steve had the genetic testing done to see if either of them carried the gene that might lead to craniosynostosis. Little did I know, but as they sat across from me at the diner and talked about their worry of having a second child, more succinctly, their worry about having a second child with craniosynostosis, Jamie was pregnant with another little guy.

I got an e-mail from Jamie the day of Evan Michael Hewitt's birth. I had been bugging her for more photos of Lucas and asking her if her new little guy had come yet. The e-mail was simple but beautiful: "Hi! He arrived today at 3:15 p.m. Has soft spots and all!! Couldn't be more thrilled!"

* * *

Sitting across from me, that same day, in the middle of one of the newest, state-of-the-art facilities for craniofacial surgery—which I was very fortunate to have Dr. Staffenberg show me around—Dr. Staffenberg clasped his hands together, leaned his elbows and forearms on his desk, and asked me if I had any more questions. This was a year before I talked to my parents about my surgery and a year before I sat down with Dr. Walker when he looked at my head and told me exactly what happened that day when they took me back into the operating room thirty-seven years earlier. I asked him what they were doing back then and, like Dr. Walker, Dr. Staffenberg told me that since it was a neurosurgeon who performed my surgery, as plastic surgeons really weren't involved much back then, they performed a strip craniectomy on me.

"What suture was closed?" he asked.

"Sagittal, I believe, based on the scar," I said. At this time, it was just a guess, as my scar traversed the sagittal line.

"Do you feel any bumps or are you pretty smooth?" he asked. His eyes concentrated on me.

"It's pretty bumpy up there and then it goes flat in the front and back," I said.

"How old were you?" he asked.

"Two months," I answered.

He sat back, straightened out his back and pulled his medical coat over his chest.

"So they either stopped the suture from fusing fully together or removed the fully fused suture. They would take silicon and actually drape it over the edges. One of the problems if removed in a baby that young, the bone may fill in again, so they would put silicon edges on the edges of the bone like this…," he said while he placed his fingers on the edges of an imaginary gap in his skull. "No matter what they did, you know, you're sort of in that fifteen percent that did fine."

I heard "fifteen percent" and questions flew into my mind. *Death? Did he mean death? Eighty-five percent died? Was I that lucky?* I managed to pull the crazy questions into one that made me seem half-intelligent.

"How would you define fifteen percent?" I asked.

"That's a great question," he said.

"On the one hand, I think we have to look at function above everything else," he said, and then paused. Then he clarified that many in the larger percentile weren't even diagnosed back then. This cleared all my previous notions about 85 percent losing their lives, as many during the early seventies were missed. My blood pressure dropped back down, but the sweat had already been released. "So what are the bad things that could have developed from craniosynostosis? Blindness, hearing problems, intellectual impairment, developmental delays, so not having those is certainly one measure of success. [With treatment] … another measure of success is the head shape. If the treatment failed and the problem didn't increase cranial pressure then the failure of the result is going to be continued narrowing and elongation of the skull."

I made a dumb joke when I left Dr. Staffenberg's office, and I felt like a complete idiot for doing so. He held the door open for me, and when I passed through I brought up what he had told me about the only 15 percent success rate. I have never been good at ending conversations, lingering on the edges of encounters far too long, as some of the families I have interviewed can attest to: we had a great conversation, but, somehow, I did a good job making the good-byes awkward. It's one of those hidden talents I have: wrapping up a good conversation with an awkward moment.

"My older brother doesn't think I was part of the fifteen percent," I said, trying to break the ice by saying that my brother felt like I had mental disabilities. Once the words left my mouth, I knew it was a boneheaded thing to say. Dr. Staffenberg, a man who had opened his doors to me and who had spent all of his professional career trying to make children's lives better, stood in front of me with no smile on his face. He understood the joke; I just do not think he understood why I would say it. Dr. Staffenberg, along with many other craniofacial surgeons, opens up children's skulls for a living, and when these surgeons are not performing surgery they are researching how to perform surgery better so the success rate will someday reach 100 percent. They see the scared families who walk into their offices. They see the family members' faces and the horror that takes them over. The surgeons have to come out into the waiting room and talk to worried families, and sometimes they have to tell families if there are any complications or down the line if there needs to be another surgery because something didn't go as well as they thought it would. And I made a dumb joke to break the awkwardness of good-byes.

A kind man, Dr. Staffenberg gave me a little smile and said, "That's what big brothers are for." The door shut behind me and the cold wind of the January in New York City splashed across my face along with my humiliation.

I walked back toward the East River for a moment and sat back down on my bench seat. In the last hour the brick promenade that led to the waving flags of the UN building had gotten even busier, but I felt completely alone. The 15 percent discussion, even though I had made a stupid joke about it, had begun to saturate my thoughts. Rarely, in my life, have I truly assessed what happened to me as an infant; rarely have I really thought about the chances that I may not have made it through or might have made it through but with a severe mental disability. That day when I sat down on the bench and watched the ferries pass in front of me and the seagulls drop down from the sky and onto the posts, for one of the first times in my life, I felt special. "Special" may not be the right word. Lucky. But I don't know if that is the right word either. I sat there as runners flew by, and as the sun began to warm my face, I felt alive, and I felt aware of my own existence and the possibility of a nonexistence or a different existence all at the same time. I'd taken it all for granted. I never really thought that I could be any different or that the risks of death or mental disabilities really applied to me. The 15 percent number was just one that Dr. Staffenberg threw out there. The number may have been higher. It probably was higher, but that doesn't matter. It was a lot lower a number than I had ever thought it to be. And I, luckily and specially, was part of it. I felt my heart beat, and as if it had pumped more blood to my skull, I swear I could feel my scar pulse up and down from the crown of my head to the back of my skull. I was truly aware of how I was born, where I came from, and how lucky I was to live such a full life and be able to walk down to the East River and watch the water drift back and forth in front of me.

Instead of taking a taxi back to our hotel near Times Square, I decided to walk. The sun had come out in full force and sat above the skyscrapers of the city. Cloudy and dizzy and awestruck from the information I had just digested, I made my way back to the hotel, crossing the street when others crossed, following the crowds, watching the feet in front of me as the crowds grew larger and larger as we got closer to the touristy square. Looking back, I barely remember the walk and I am surprised I had enough sense to make it to the hotel, following the street signs, and not get hit by a car.

PART SIX: FAULT LINES (SAGITTAL SYNOSTOSIS)

The Plains

It was one of those roads that make you wonder if you are in the right place, in the right city, on the right path. I headed north of Kansas City and passed Saint Joseph, a town that from the freeway looked tired, with red faded brick buildings and empty roads. And the city passed beside me like years that I had no memory of, a glimpse into something that I could only place in my mind as a photo, those when I was bandaged and bruised and swollen and swaddled in my parents' arms. Recently, my mom has shared baby photos of me, opened up dusty and yellowing photo spreads and handed them to me to look at. Many of them I had never seen before. She has handed them to me or sent them to me as scans, but she doesn't say anything more than, "You were a beautiful boy from the moment I laid eyes on you." That's all she allows herself to let go before moving onto another conversation. I know my mom, and I know that she would never hide the photos or be ashamed of them or me as a baby. She's told me a million times over the years that I was a beautiful baby even with my skull pointed forward and backward like a falling cone. There are photos, two or three of them, of me leaning backward on a nearly fluorescent seventies multi-colored striped chair at my grandma's house. The elongated shape of my skull, doing its best to grow, drops a shadow on the chair. The shadow is not rounded or oval but pointy. Then, as if the next photo was taken a moment later, I am propped up more and turned a little sideways. It looks like my parents were taking mug shots of me, but I'm guessing they wanted to capture an image of their boy before the surgery that would open his skull came around the corner of their twenty-something-year-old lives and took me away—just like the memory of every parent I have spoken with, the last thoughts before the nurse took their child away remain the most powerful of any, even for those tough parents who were strong.

But, as I write this, it is all speculative, saving my mom from a long conversation until the end of this journey when I can finish the book and send it off and we can be done with it for a while. In the next photo, my dad has picked me up and cradled me in his arms. The blur of my head shows that I was crying and bucking in his arms, but his big, young hands and fingers wrap nearly all the way around my little torso, capturing all my movement in, for him, a tiny squeeze. The next photo in the pile shows me in a bandage after surgery, my turban, as my parents called it, and the description is accurate. The white cloth wraps around the forehead and above my ears and extends upward above my head five or six inches. The upper layer of gauze and cloth holds in layers of blood and other, more deliberate bandaging that covers my incisions and newly shaped skull. And then the baby photos become toddler photos with my blond and white-shaded hair growing over my skull and the scar taking on the duties of a part down the middle and pushing my hair to the sides.

I drive northward toward a little town named Amazonia, the world of a young childhood that I can't even imagine flies by me like the mile signs on Interstate 29, and I head to see a little boy who, like me, was born with sagittal synostosis, the first child I would meet with the same closed suture as me, and for some reason that can't be explained without using the words "silly" or "nonsensical" or "without reason" I am nervous to meet the little boy and his parents, to walk into their home and say hello, and to be somewhat of a fortune-teller of what their son will end up like. What if I disappointed them, left them hoping that their son will turn out better, smarter, or easier around people, that he wouldn't act too nervous around new people, be too polite, or maybe, and the silliest thought of them all, that he will be much taller than his sagittal predecessor?

The buildings and homes become sporadic and gaps of Missouri countryside that are covered with the brown tall grass of winter become larger and larger until there are no more McDonald's or Burger Kings or gas stations. A two-lane highway weaves away from Interstate 29, and I follow it until I reach the beaten-up town of Amazonia. Rusty trailer homes and slumping foundations seem to grow out of the landscape like deteriorating caves. The road heads farther out into the country and parallels train tracks until County Road 409 finally appears and leads me over the tracks and onto a dirt road that has become mostly mud after the recent snowstorm that gave Kansas City and Wichita the most inches in recorded history for the month of February 2013.

Mary and I had sold our Jeep a few years back and replaced it with a Hyundai, and at that moment when the front two wheels spun out a bit I wished we hadn't sold the Jeep. The muddy road ascended Missouri's hilly terra. The wheels slipped back and forth, got traction and straightened out, slipped back and forth again and got traction until we, my little Hyundai and I, crested the hill and wiggled our way through the muddy landscape and sat in the driveway of the DeVooghts. Snow covered their lawn and, like I always do, I waited in the car for a minute to gather myself. I'm not good at meeting new people, so I have to dig down into myself, breathe long and deep breaths, and calm the nervous hands that twist and squeeze my intestines.

Aimee met me outside with a warm smile and a finger that pointed me toward a path of footprints that had been made by her husband when he jumped out of his car in his work boots and plodded toward the garage door entrance. I wore nice shoes and a collared shirt, hoping, again, that as I stood in front of them as a full-time instructor at Kansas State University they would see that there were, I hoped, no mental setbacks from the early closure and release of my sagittal suture. I've never thought of myself as an academic. I admit in most social circles when asked why I don't have a PhD and how I landed such a good teaching gig that I just don't have the mind of an academic, that I'm an artist, and that I truly don't believe I have a PhD kind of brain, which I truly believe. Most of the time people think I should be smarter than I am or that I should carry myself in that academic way people see in the movies or remember from their collegiate years, the well-spoken, extremely well-read teacher who never stumbles over words and always says the right thing; that is not me. I live in a pool of stumbled words, awkward comments, and saying the exact wrong thing. That day, on the way to the DeVooght's, for some silly reason, I wanted to seem as smart as I possibly could. I wanted them to see the moment Aimee stepped out in the snow to meet me that I was of at least average intelligence and that her son, Wyatt, could be very, very smart—in my mind, much smarter than me.

When I saw Wyatt for the first time, he jumped and bounced around the house. He smiled like any three-year-old-boy would. He gave off a warmth that filled the room and made his parents roll their eyes at his openness to strangers. Two minutes into my visit, he began to crawl on me and grab my hand in an attempt to show me his room. He climbed on the table and sat between his mom Aimee and me, and his dad rolled his eyes in a way that only parents can, saying in one shift of his brow, *This little guy of mine is rambunctious, sitting on the table, and although I should be angry, everything in me wants to laugh because I love him so much.* I know that eye roll because Lukas makes me do it many times a day.

Wyatt was the first sagittal boy I have, knowingly, ever met in my life, and when I shifted him from one chair to the other when he attempted to climb through me all I could think about was, *I'm a sagittal cranio boy, and I am honored to be in the company of a Wyatt and all the rest.*

The conversation took a minute to roll out, and like many parents choose to do, Aimee started with pictures. Pictures break down walls—they are a gift to me, a brave gift to welcome me in. Little Wyatt's pre-surgery head was bulbous, extending outward on the sides, his frozen sagittal suture making the path for his brain limited. His little eyes sat beneath his extending forehead. He looked like a sagittal boy, the most common of the craniosynostosis children. But his smile matched that of the little boy who climbed on me like I was a mobile playground, a naturally sweet boy.

"I knew something was wrong immediately," Aimee said. Her husband sat across from me and nodded his head in quiet agreement. Aimee talked about Wyatt's cranial vault remodeling. The doctors opened him up, pulled Wyatt's skull off of his head from the brow upward, purposely cracked and chiseled at his bone, removed the synosed suture, and then remodeled his skull, doing everything necessary to place the bone back together in the most effective structural and growth patterns as well as the most aesthetically pleasing manner that would match what most believe is a nicely shaped head.

The CVR technique for correcting the fusion of the sagittal suture, as well as the endoscopic techniques, are the most commonly used techniques today, as the endoscopic techniques, according to many surgeons, are most effective in children under three months of age. Any older than that and many surgeons, including Dr. Staffenberg, Dr. Fearon, and Dr. Walker, believe a full CVR is the best way to correct the sagittal suture and reshape the skull.

Dr. Staffenberg, in his office that day in NYC, talked about why a full CVR is better for the older children with sagittal synostosis:

> In babies, the missing bone will gradually fill in on its own. For you and I, if somebody removes that bone, it will never fill in again, but in babies it would, and so you can imagine from that there's some sort of time limit that if we leave more time, eventually, that [endoscopy] won't work anymore. In other words, if we have a child who's fully grown, and we do that and put a molding helmet on, their brain is grown, there's no force anymore to push the head to the side, so it's a technique that we consider mainly in younger babies and at some point we believe that the efficacy of that [endoscopy] technique starts to diminish and that the greatest likelihood of success, in our opinion, is in babies that are no more than three months old.
>
> There are definitely exceptions, but there are surgeons who have a single operation that they do and that's the operation that they do. We'd rather sort of think of each baby individually ... if we're going to do an operation, we're committed to getting the best possible results. If we feel that a larger operation is necessary because the chances that the simpler operation getting a good

result are smaller, then we're only going to be doing a larger operation if it gives us a return on that investment.

It's our job to make sure that we're doing it in a way that it's going to be safe, you know? You want to get where you're going and you don't want to be late. You might have to drive a little faster, as long as you're within the speed limit, but it goes without saying that you want to be safe also—so that's our job. Our job is to do it with whatever considerations are necessary to make the operation as safe as possible, but the reason that we make an operation more complicated is only to increase our chances of getting the outcome that we want and minimize the chances that we would need to do something more.

Dr. Staffenberg explained that for sagittal synostosis, with the elongated and narrow head where the middle suture has closed up, for a baby who is six months or older the question becomes: How do we fix that child's skull shape? "Well, we could certainly do the same thing and put a helmet on. The helmet is not under my control, you know, so in a sense, when we do the strip craniectomy, at the end of the operation baby's head is the same shape, baby's skull is the same shape. If we get some improvement in shape, it's because of the helmet. It's not because of anything that I'm doing," he answers his question, and explains that a full CVR may entail more risk and may take longer, but if it's going to prevent another surgery it is a better investment in time. Maybe the scar will be longer, and he notes that others may judge him on that, but his view is that if a larger scar in this situation will give better results then it is worth it in the long run of the child's life.

The relationship between the neurosurgeon and plastic surgeon changes, evolves, and is different within each team, and this relationship is extremely important. Most of the time, the neurosurgeon makes the initial incisions and removes the skull so the plastic surgeon can reshape the skull. The neurosurgeon provides the safest access to that very important part of a child's anatomy and sometimes the roles between neurosurgeon and plastic surgeon within the craniofacial team can be murky, but each team works that out on their own.

Dr. Staffenberg, with a set of surgical photos in front of him from his recent publication, explained the procedure for a sagittal CVR:

So if we were looking at sort of profile view of the child's head, and here's the nose and chin here, we would be removing say something like this [he points to the area of skull removed]. So all of this now is still not a brain operation because we're outside the dura. It's only the bone that we're removing and we can now take the bone on the side. The part of the bone where the suture is, is not used in the reconstruction, but the rest of the bone is otherwise normal bone and we can use that to make a new occiput, or the part of the bone in the back of the skull, and we can put that on here. And then another piece of bone, we can actually put along the top of the head and all of this is held with little dissolving plates and screws, so that this then becomes a very solid unit, so immediately after the operation a baby can lie down on the back of their head, but by sort of shifting this forward the brain actually pushes out on the side and so the shape of the head then becomes shorter from front to back and wider on the side, which is the head shape that we want. By the end of the operation, we have that head shape established. And then the side areas, we use remaining piece of the bone that we can actually split into an inner layer and an outer layer and bone graft these areas so this sort of becomes a mosaic of bone and that bone heals just like any other broken bone, so that a few weeks later, when they come back to the office, the parents even say, when they wash the baby's hair, they say it now feels like a normal skull. It's unlike using, say, titanium or artificial bone. The baby's own bone, remember, is designed from the beginning to grow with the brain underneath pushing it [the skull], so this bone has the ability not to just heal or fuse, but it has the ability to what we say "remodel." It gradually, as the brain is pushing underneath, the inner layer of the bone will gradually be dissolved by the body and new bone is deposited on the outer layer and so the normal dynamic of bone growth is continuing but without that new suture.

While Wyatt's surgeons and other surgeons using the CVR techniques across the country may have done things a little differently, the basic tenets of the CVR are very common.

* * *

Aimee laughed and chatted, her husband sitting quietly next to her.

"I don't know," she said. "I think I should have been more worried about the whole thing, but I wasn't. Does that make me a bad mother?" She laughed a bit more and hugged Wyatt some more.

"I mean, everything went well; everything was okay," she said. The DeVooghts' house, their older teenage daughter dressed in a cheerleading outfit, was calm. To be honest, that was the exact way Aimee should have felt with the advancements of surgical treatment to treat craniosynostosis, especially with how common the revaulting of sagittal synostosis has become. When Wyatt was opened up in 2009, it had been more than fifty (or more) years since the morbidity rate and rate of complications were high. All parents who have a child born with craniosynostosis in this day and age should feel assured that their child will be safe and that the surgery will go well. We are very far from the days of surgical worry or uncertainty, but this is not something that can be told to a mother and father who must hand the child over to have his or her head opened up and reconstructed, but Aimee had it right; she believed in her doctor, her surgeon, and the advancement of surgical technology, and no it didn't make her a bad mother because she didn't worry more, just as worrying horribly doesn't make other mothers bad moms either. It just made her

Wyatt's mother, the calm, loving mother who would take him to and from the hospital and watch him climb all over without a worry for his head.

I left the DeVooughts' house, tromped through the late-spring snow, and drove my Hyundai down the dirt road to meet a stopped train on the tracks. I sat and thought about Aimee's words and about how she hadn't been as worried as some other mothers I had encountered over more than two years of research, and I thought, *Soon enough, when enough people know about this common birth defect and the commonality of the surgical procedures to correct it, they will, hopefully, feel that way too.*

A train sat in front of me at the end of the dirt road that led away from the DeVooghts' home, stalled in my pathway back to Manhattan, Kansas, a two-hour drive that I really wanted to get started on late that evening, but the cold air sat on my windshield and battled against my defroster until I rolled down the window and let the chill fall into the front seat of my little car and I breathed out for the first time that night knowing that I didn't have to prove anything to this loving family. They already had what they needed. With the cold air in my lungs, I laughed at the idea that at one time I thought I needed to prove anything.

The Apparatus (Endoscopy and Helmet Therapy)

Camille (Calli) Rhoades, mother of Xaida Rhoades, saw the old man from across the local supermarket. He stared at the helmet on Xaida's head, his eyes focusing in on the not-yet-one- year-old girl whose helmet, covered in stickers and artwork, enveloped most of her head. The transparent, thick plastic that dropped down all the way to her brow, ran over her temples, around her ears, and back down to the base of her neck must have rattled him, because he had obviously forgotten that watching strangers in a supermarket and making an, albeit very slow, beeline across the floor would not be seen as well mannered. But Calli spotted him as he walked toward them in the aisle. She saw his raised eyebrow and squinting eyes, his mind spinning around the little girl with the helmet.

Calli braced herself for what was to come. She knew something "good," as she puts it, was on its way. The man moved his head around. He scanned the helmet, almost ignoring the little girl beneath it, and stopped and stared.

"I've never seen an apparatus on a child like that before," he said. "What kind of apparatus is this?"

Calli dove into explanations of craniosynostosis and began to discuss her child's surgery, but the old man didn't bring his eyes up to meet Calli's eyes. He just continued to stare at the apparatus and then moved on, satisfied enough in the knowledge that the apparatus actually existed, not needing to know why.

The old man in the supermarket was not alone in his curiosity. Xaida's helmet caught the attention of children too, and like the old man who had no need to filter his curiosity, children, as their curiosity naturally gets the best of them and takes over their mouths, could not hold in their questions.

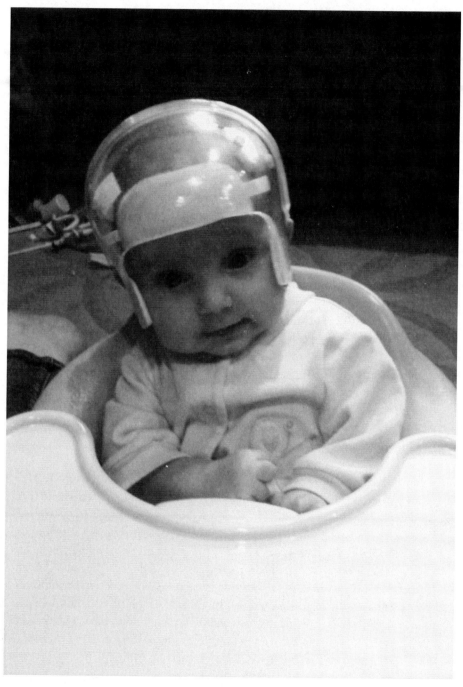

Helmet therapy with endoscopic surgery (courtesy of Camille Rhoades).

Shocked mothers winced and smiled uncomfortable smiles when Calli and Xaida stood behind them at the store or walked by them at church. The mothers knew that there would be no stopping their little ones from pointing at the little girl.

"What's wrong with your baby's head?" the kids would ask, their mothers gasping and grabbing their children's arms to bring down the pointer fingers. Calli, however, and despite the pure embarrassment of the mothers of the kids, didn't mind telling them that when Xaida was born her head didn't form right, so the doctors had to fix it and put the helmet on her to protect her until she got better. Kids were happy with that, and the finger-pointing went away.

Old men and children get a pass.

As most mothers know and as my wife can attest, adults—mainly women—forget they are strangers when they see a pregnant woman in public. They stalk and stare. They position themselves like roadblocks in front of the expecting mother, they ask, out of nowhere, when the baby is due, without the slightest introduction, but worst of all, some will walk up to the mother, place their hands on her belly, and rub without permission. Calli and Xaida got to continue on with this tradition long after Xaida was born.

"Why does she have that?" and "What's the helmet for?" and "What's wrong with her head?" came from the mouths of complete strangers, blowing the minds of Calli and her husband. The sheer number of strangers who approached them and bluntly asked these questions made Xaida's parents laugh out loud when I spoke with them. Most mothers asked if it was because she had a misshapen head, positional plagiocephaly, and out of the need to answer if they felt the need to question Calli explained Xaida's craniosynostosis, the need for surgery, and the importance of the helmet.

At other times, well-intentioned baby lovers walked up behind Xaida's baby carrier, Xaida tucked into it like a precious nut in a squirrel's hand, her and her helmet hidden from sight. The baby lovers leaned their heads around the edges of the baby carrier and peered in to look at Xaida. They did not expect to see the helmet. They couldn't hide their surprise. Some people let out vocal expressions of their surprise by gasping or saying, "Oooh." Others, incapable of controlling their physical reaction, snapped their neck and head backward, and their eyes spread open like an egg dropping into a frying pan, the yolk big and yellow in the center of expanding whiteness. They could barely see Xaida within the helmet, but most were very kind.

"She's so darling," they'd say. "She's so darling in that helmet, though," they'd tell Calli, doing their best to recover from their fried-egg eyes.

"She's darling, for sure, but I just wished people saw past the helmet and the need to say 'in that helmet.'" Calli laughed out loud. "'Why does she have to wear that thing?'"

In the end, though, Calli and Dustin felt the helmet gave them the chance to explain the birth defect to legitimately interested people at church, at school, and at work. When children are born with multi-sutural fusion, sagittal fusion most commonly makes up one of the fused sutures, which partly accounts for the high number of sagittal cases. Xaida, like many children with sagittal craniosynostosis, had a partially fused suture. It had closed up but not all of the way, leaving a tiny anterior fontanel.

"She has a soft spot," the Rhoadeses' pediatrician told them when he scanned Xaida's head at her two-week appointment, "but it's about the size of the tip of my finger." While sagittal sutures may only be partially closed at birth, the birth defect may or may not continue to close prematurely throughout the first few years of child's life, so there is no way of assessing the extent of the damage to the brain or the extent of the malformation of the skull at such an early age. Some within the medical community believe that partial sagittal craniosynostosis is a type of craniosynostosis that lends itself to the option of nonsurgical repair or no repair at all—most do not believe this— even though doctors are pressured to tell families that the surgery is optional, the medical community believes that there really is no option besides surgical reconstruction of the cranium to free the suture and therefore free the brain to grow.

Dr. Staffenberg warns about leaving a partially closed suture to run its course:

> It's going to finish its job. It'll finish its job, and I think that's the way we have to think about it to be successful. What we cannot predict yet with 100 percent accuracy is how rapidly it will progress. In other words, that suture is going to fuse like a zipper, but how fast is that zipper going to close? And we also can't predict, if left alone, how severe the changes will be by the time the child is finished growing, so a lot of babies now will come to me with more mild forms, mild changes. Everyone's getting a little bit more sensitized to the entity of craniosynostosis because of, you know, books and Web sites that are out there and so they'll come in and they'll, you know, I'll see a baby with very mild changes and it's a little bit like seeing the photograph of a race car on a track. You know that the race car is moving because the background is blurry, but if somebody asked you, "How fast is that race car going?" you wouldn't be able to tell them.

Since treating craniosynostosis enables the brain to expand and the brain to grow, pushing the skull outward, surgery is suggested by most surgeons; however, when multiple sutures are closed there are fewer options, as the chances of "mental impairment" and blindness rise drastically when two or more sutures are closed (pancraniosysnostosis). Since Xaida only had one fused suture, her doctor needed to present the family with the most common options available today.

Months before the helmet had been placed on Xaida's head, Calli held her baby's head in her hand as her body lay in a pink tub of warm water that cradled her arms and legs. Her face shone bright red, still bruised from labor, and her head lay softly in her mother's hands. Her forehead rose up from her brow and the top of her head flatly fell backward until it reached her anterior fontanel and then dropped with a drastic angle downward toward her neck. From her neck up, it looked as if her skull was molded around a raw bean.

"It is amazing to me to think that we didn't realize there was a problem. It is SO clear there [looking at a photo of Xaida's first bath]. I just had no frame of reference to think there was anything to worry about," Calli said. The CT scan of Xaida's head shows the partial closure of the sagittal suture. From the posterior fontanel it stretches clean and open toward the front of Xaida's head but then closes off like a riverbed that dried up before it could reach its destination, the anterior fontanel. The space on the skull where the suture should remain open lay smooth and dense and hardened. By the time the surgery day approached, Xaida's head had elongated, her brain and skull filling up the back part of bean-shaped bone. A head cloth had been placed over Xaida's head the day of surgery so she could receive blood work and another scan. The white cloth accentuated the elongated length of the back of her skull; the edge of the white cloth contrasted against the pink skin, and like an artist sketching the edges of an upcoming work, the cloth illustrated the irregular skull shape, not letting the eye follow the skin from the top of the skull to the neck but outlining the deformation.

Beyond the stretching of the back of the skull, the colliding plates of Xaida's head created a massive (for a child's head) ridge at the top of her head, like the two tectonic plates slamming into each with nowhere to go but up, but instead of giant mountains of rock shooting upward, Xaida's skull rose to a jagged ridge where her sagittal suture should have remained open.

Calli, sitting with the doctor and Dustin just a few days after Xaida's birth, was given four options, and for her as a mother options were her worst enemy, begging her to answer the question, "What is best for my child?," pushing her to look into the future and predict long-term outcomes, forcing her to confront her own beliefs about what is important in the life of a child, of a teen, of a young adult, and, way down the line, an adult.

The neurosurgeon sat Calli and Dustin down.

A nice man with a nice, calming way about him, he gave them three options.

First, he talked about the option of not having surgery and the benefits and the risks of what that option carried: Some believe that there are great risks of the development of mental disabilities, while others believe there is very little risk in this case, "Without the surgery, your child may be a physicist, when she could have been an astrophysicist," the neurosurgeon explained. This conclusion that there might be a higher chance of a learning disability in those who elect not to have cranial surgery in single-suture sagittal craniosynostosis has been, for the most part, anecdotal, physicians recognizing an increase in learning disabilities and cognitive problems in those not electing surgery, because an extensive study on those with untreated cranioysynostis has been nearly impossible to conduct. Xaida's doctor gave them the best, most appropriate answer based on studies up until that point, as most babies with single suture sagittal craniosynostosis have corrective surgery and there is no definitive research to prove the higher chance of neuropsychological or psychosocial effects on these children.

"This is the only time we're going to use this word," their doctor said to them. "But this surgery could be considered cosmetic." The words came from his mouth, and although the Rhoadeses had already decided that Xaida would have surgery, the use of the word "cosmetic" spun them a little, planting that morsel of doubt in their mind and making them ask again, "Is this surgery for us or is it for our daughter?" The word "cosmetic" gets tossed around a lot when it comes to partial-sagittal reconstruction, because the science isn't there to prove the developmental repercussions of not having surgical care and a large part of the surgery involves reshaping the baby's head to be aesthetically pleasing, as doctors could open up the skull, fix the problem, close it up, and not worry about beveling and shaping and forming a nice-looking skull. So, the word "cosmetic" throws a weird kink into the decision process for parents. It makes them doubt their intentions. It makes them wonder if their needs are shallow, but the Rhoadeses, not wanting to take a chance on the mental development of their child, accepted that they were also making the decision to, they hoped, stave off abnormal psychological development by eliminating the chance of Xaida growing up different. If they could do both, they no longer would doubt their decision.

"Plus, children and people are cruel," Dustin said. "Kids are cruel. We knew, having raised three other children before Xaida, that a lot more goes into a child's development than just what happens on the inside of the skull. We knew that if she looked different and we had the chance to help avoid verbal abuse we would do it in a heartbeat."

The second option the neurosurgeon discussed was endoscopic surgery to correct the fused suture. He discussed the option thoroughly, noting the benefits of the less invasive procedure, the less time in the PICU and the lesser use of blood transfusion. Over the last thirty-five years, beginning just a few years after my surgery in 1976, surgical techniques had evolved rapidly and led the way for less invasive surgeries, surgeries that do not involve full cranial vault reconstruction and remodeling. These techniques have shown to be very successful, not only in the less invasive removal of bone but also in the reshaping of the skull to be aesthetically pleasing. Drs. David F. Jimenez and Constance M. Barone pushed toward the use of endoscopy and back toward the strip craniotomy that had been nearly abandoned since the years before and during my surgical procedure. Jimenez and Barone reintroduced the shaping helmet, brought about in the 1980s, that had also fallen out of favor. When Calli's doctor brought up the need for the shaping helmet and how Xaida would have to wear it for nearly a year post-surgery, Calli was taken back a bit, worried about a full year of the stares and questions and awkwardness the helmet would indefinitely bring about.

There has been research, however, on the elevated chances of neuropsychological and psychosocial effects, as well as learning disabilities and cognitive problems, on a large sampling of children who had less invasive surgery to correct their fused suture, therefore eliminating any type of cognitive problems due to "limited bone removal and little chance for brain damage during surgery." This type of research would relate directly to the second option the doctor gave the Rhoadeses that afternoon.

The doctor gave the Rhoadeses two other options, both involving much more invasive cranial surgery, such as a full CVR.

"As a parent, you want so badly to make the right decisions. And no one can make those decisions for you. You want so badly to make the right ones, and as a parent, I am always second-guessing myself," said Calli. "I wondered, what if I don't make the right decision? What if something goes wrong and I can't go back? What if this is about me? What if I mess up my kid?" The what ifs that plague all the parents who face this decision because the words "optional" and "cosmetic" are lofted into the air by medical professionals who have to say them for liability reasons. Almost like speaking to future parents who will face this decision, Calli continued, her voice rising in pitch and strength, her hands coming down onto her knees and her upper body leaning forward like a quarterback calling out the last desperation play of game, "You can't do that. I have to go with my gut. With my prayers."

The Rhoadeses walked into the meeting with the doctor having already made a decision to put their daughter under the knife, but after listening to what was said during the meeting they both felt differently. "You have to let go; you have to accept that you are going to let someone you don't know cut open your child's head. And it is so scary." Calli, a women who smiles more than she frowns, whose laughter leaves her easily and steadily and with no effort, choked up when talking about her fears. Her laughter left her for five minutes when she talked about the decision, when, obviously, the moment the doctors took her daughter away swam through her memory. Then the laughter came again when the memories swam away and the reality that her daughter made it through came back.

Dustin had made up his mind before he left the doctor's office. He knew that endoscopy was the best option for Xaida, and most within the field would agree that Xaida was an excellent candidate for endoscopic treatment. But Calli struggled with it, consulting other parents who had two children with craniosynostosis, the first child having the larger-scale surgery to release the fused suture and the other having the endoscopic surgery, and was surprised at what the other parents told her: the other parents described the lumpiness and scars of the older child and the relatively less physical evidence of the endoscopic surgery. This, to Calli, seemed counterintuitive. In her mind, she had expected to hear the opposite. She had expected to hear that the endoscopic surgery had less successful results. The less invasive surgery screamed out to her to be a shortcut method to "fix" her child's skull. Unlike her husband, she struggled with the decision, defining her struggle as that of a mom's worry.

Another mother who faced the same disheartening, gut-wrenching, life-altering diagnosis for not only one but both of her children told Calli her story, revealing her own doubts about the endoscopic method to release the suture: the mother walked into the recovery room post-surgery and felt like the doctors had forgotten to operate on her second child. She had feared the day of her second child's surgery, remembering the scarring and swelling after the opening up and reconstructing of her first child's sutures, so when she walked into the post-operative room and saw the minimal swelling and puffiness, she worried the doctors hadn't done what they needed to do, but after recovery the baby was fine, was better than fine; he recovered with much more ease than her first child, who had gone through a more severe cranial vault.

After talking to those parents and listening to their stories, Calli felt confident in the decision that her husband had found the day in the doctor's office: endoscopic surgery to release the sagittal suture.

* * *

Drs. David F. Jimenez and Constance M. Barone are considered by many to be the pioneers of endoscopic surgery to release the fused sutures of the skull. Their techniques found what many have found since when using endoscopic techniques: less blood loss, less time in the operating room, less expensive hospital costs, and less time in the hospital post-surgeries. To many, these two doctors are seen as the revivalists of the strip craniotomy and endoscopic surgery for treatment of craniosynostosis, as they do very little reconstruction when releasing the suture, opening the skull, grafting the fused bone, making sure there is no closure, closing the child back up again, and fitting them for a helmet that does a lot of the reconstruction.

Endoscopic surgical procedures, like full-cranial vault procedures, vary based on the doctor's experience and preferred technique; however, the variance between endoscopic procedures can be seen as much less than between its more invasive counterparts.

Most current endoscopic reconstruction research, researchers, doctors, and clinical studies point to the initial work and documentation of Drs. Jimenez and Barone; they dove into the deep end of the pool when they began relieving the closed sutures of craniosynostosis in the mid–1990s. Endoscopic surgery, having been used in numerous types of surgeries for decades—even centuries if one counts the early uses of primitive endoscopes to look at the human abdomen—has been proven to lead the way in minimally invasive surgery (MIS), and the technology rapidly advanced in the 1990s. As proof, I tore my ACL in 1991. In 1992 I had a full reconstructive surgery that failed just weeks post-op, despite opening up my knee and leaving a nine-inch scar from quadriceps to shin. One year later I had another surgery to repair the busted ligament, this time endoscopically repaired, leaving only two tiny incision marks, and twenty years later I have a well-repaired knee, so it was at the same time that Jimenez and Barone began researching and performing cranial-based endoscopic repairs.

In 1996 Jimenez and Barone began using endoscopes to fix sagittal synostosis in four infants. Since then, up to 2012, they have treated 256 infants, and the results were very successful and the long-term results were just as successful, not having to perform more surgeries for correction. Of those infants, more than two-thirds were male, as other studies have shown the prominence of synostosis in males and even a higher prominence of sagittal synostosis in males, and the average age was just under four months, and all infants were placed in molding helmets post-surgery—Jimenez and Barone used the cephalic index, a measurement to calculate the breadth of skull by centimeters to judge head shape based on length—and 87 percent were classified as excellent, 9 percent were classified as good, and 4 percent were classified as poor. The doctors found that their method, one that varies little from surgeon to surgeon, presented fantastic results with "minimal morbidity and complications and improved results over traditional procedures." Jimenez and Barone felt that the best patients for this MIS are children under the age of three months because young infants handle the surgery very well, the calvarial bone, the skull, is still very thin, and the deploe, the spongy and porous space between the outer skull and the inner skull and the deploic space, is small, lending to the surgery causing less blood loss. Since the calvaria is thin and the brain grow so rapidly at this age, the marrying of the two typically leads to a natural correction of the affected area. The doctors believe that children between the ages of three and six months are still good candidates, but because of the natural thickening of the skull bone and chances of more blood loss the surgery becomes more complicated. After six months of age, however, this technique becomes much more complicated and children with severe malformation of the skull are no longer deemed plausible candidates for the procedure.

Some doctors scan the skull with their hands, like reading a diagnosis in braille. The bumps of bone talk to them and tell them history of the baby's cranium, how it developed, and if the sutures prematurely ossified. Some doctors, like the Ehmanns' doctor in Denver, do not usually use CT scans at all in determining if the baby was born with craniosynostosis, some begin with a CT scan, and others use it as a supplement to physical cranial analysis. Once the situation is assessed, however, and the decision is made by the parents, surgery follows.

A year before I talked with the Rhoades family, Xaida's head was prepped for surgery with a povidone-iodine solution, a solution commonly used in move invasive surgeries to fight off possible infections. Jimenez and Barone's technique has changed little over the years, and in 2012 and in recent years prior to 2012 they added new instruments to the procedure to help with visualization of the interior of the scalp and help keep the internal environment of the body stable (homeostasis). In the case of endoscopic surgery for the reconstruction of the fused sagittal suture, according to Drs. Jimenez and Barone in their publication "Endoscopic Technique for Sagittal Synostosis," published in the journal *Childs Nervous System*, "a general examination is done and any comorbidities are properly addressed, the patient may be taken for surgery. We do not routinely obtain extensive blood work and only get a heel stick hematocrit once the patient is under general anesthesia. There is no need for arterial, central venous lines or a Foley catheter." Special bone-cutting instruments and dural retractors are used to help cauterize the diploie, the veins and blood in the diploic space (the space between the two layers of bone in the skull).

Then the child is put in the sphinx position. Her neck is extended forward and prepped for the upcoming incisions. In other words, with the baby in the sphinx position, the endotracheal tube, the tube used to help the baby breathe, is placed into baby's mouth and nose and extended into the trachea to ensure breathing. (I imagine these children stretched out like dolls on a factory floor as the factory workers extend and shift the children's bodies to add pieces to fill an order. Their necks fall downward toward the floor, and their hands extend out beneath them.) Jinenez and Barone anesthesiologist has put the infant to sleep and the baby's skull waits for the first incision. Before the first incision, Jimenez and Barone don't typically do extensive blood work on the child, opting to only take blood for a blood count from the heel once the child has fallen asleep, his eyes have closed and his world has gone dark. While many institutions secure an arterial line, typically in the radial artery (wrist), for the anesthesiologist to check the labs intraoperatively and monitor the blood pressure beat to beat, Jimenez and Barone do not, a preference defined by the doctors and institution. With endoscopic surgery, most institutions do not secure a central venous line, a line that is placed in the internal jugular, subclavian, or femoral veins, for the anesthesiologist to give medications that directly affect the patient's heart—these central lines, however, are very common in the classic (open) repair of synostosis because the open procedure has more blood loss. The sphinx position ensures the endotracheal tube functions properly, giving the infant's lungs a clear path for air throughout the surgery.

Then the cutting begins. The doctors' hands, typically all four of them moving together in a synchronous rhythm of fingers and palms and wrists, cut two incisions perpendicular to the midline of the skull, slicing through the skin of the child. One incision is made behind the midline and behind the anterior fontanel and the lambda. Typically, a cautery scalpel is used to cut into the pericranium, the membrane that covers the other skull (or skull periosteum), and deep into the subgaleal space, the space between the bones of the skull. Beneath the layer of skin, blood and tissue shine bright red, redder than any blood that flows out of a cut or wound of the skin. There are deep reds and nearly fluorescent reds that lie beneath the first layers of the periosteum. The contrast between skin and the redness of what lies beneath is drastic and sharp. The doctors hold scalp elevators in their hands and squeeze the hands to clamp the metal ends around the edges of skin at the incision and then peel back to reveal even more of the bright red that lies beneath. The endoscope helps to dissect the subgaleal space along with a retractor blade, a blade end shaped like the edge of an iPhone but much thinner, which elevates the scalp, and a needle tip monopolar, a device used to electrically cauterize the loose areolar tissue, unstructured tissue that surrounds blood vessels and vein. All of this helps to minimize the blood during dissection and keeps the pericranium intact.

The doctors then move the suction tip and the endoscope back and forth until they are able to make contact with the lambdoid sutures. The dura, at this point, is completely separated from the bone and the cutting of the bone, laterally and around the midline (paramedian), is made with bone-cutting scissors. Doctors must decide how much bone to cut out of the skulls, but for the most part this decision is defined by the age of the baby. The younger the child, the more bone the doctors remove, as the skull has more room to grow. In very young children, doctors will remove up to five or six centimeters of bone. As the child's age increases, the amount of centimeters of bone removed decreases to as low as two or three. Endoscopic surgery is rarely used in children above the age of six months. Children who have surgery very early will have much more bone, respectively, than, say, their five-year-old peers. The removal (cutting) of bone creates a midline strip of bone and the bone is cut again at the front of the lambdoid and behind the coronal sutures. By doing this, the surgeons give the skull the chance to grow to a shape that we see as normal (cephalic index). Surgeons at this point in the procedure do their best to create hemostasis (the lack of bleeding) in and around the bone to prevent future post-operative complications—this has been the technique of Drs. Jimenez and Barone for a lot of years. Then the child is taken away to recovery and eventually to be fitted for a custom-made helmet that will restrict growth in the front and the back of the skull and promote growth on the sides of the skull, just like Xaida's.

If, and only if, a child is a suitable candidate for endoscopic surgery (which will be at the discretion of the surgeon), the benefits of endoscopic surgery have been highly touted: there is minimal blood loss and low transfusion rates, it is well tolerated by younger infants, and the post-operative stay in the hospital is much shorter. Xaida, like many, fulfilled the criteria for endoscopic surgery, as she was young enough to have it performed and the use of endoscopic surgery to release the sagittal suture has been used, and practiced, most often, as her brother would tell you.

Xaida came out of surgery and had a bit of trouble breathing the first day but overcame this problem quickly. Her dark hair had been shaved from her forehead to the first scar that lay perpendicular to her sagittal suture, then more hair; then parallel to the first incision lay her second incision like an island in a sea of dark brown hair. The incisions, unlike the zigzag from ear to ear typically left from more invasive surgery, one of the options for Xaida and the only option for other children, are clean and straight. Xaida's incisions are small. They run parallel to each other, one in the center of the skull and the second toward the back. Her light blond hair lies over them, and they are light pink, the harsh red faded from them. Her curls cover them up as she bounces around the couch and harasses her older siblings, but they cuddle her and play with her and giggle at her two-year-old eccentricities. The scars are not part of their daily playtime.

She blossomed every day, crying less and smiling more, but when she was ten weeks old, after the surgery, the doubts invaded Calli. Helmet day sucked. Helmet day created the doubt about their choice of surgery she had been able to avoid until that point. They placed the helmet on Xaida's head and tightened the Velcro down, the sound of Velcro that would make the baby cry when she heard it.

"Did we make the right decision?" Calli asked herself over and over again on helmet day. "Should we have just done the longer, bigger surgery and just walked out with it all done?" she asked herself the first few weeks while strapping the stinky plastic helmet down onto Xaida's head with Velcro. Even in the cold Utah winter when Xaida got her helmet, the heat from her head clouded up the air beneath the plastic. The year ahead with the helmet looked like it would never end. It looked like an insurmountable challenge that Calli and Dustin just didn't know if they could tackle, strapping hard plastic to their child's head every day and leaving it there for twenty-three out of twenty-four hours so it could help the baby's head and skull grow, giving her brain room to expand without slamming into hard bone.

At that time, they doubted their choice and wondered if they had made a mistake. But when Xaida adjusted to it, as did her parents, looking down at her daughter, Calli hoped that she would be "just cute enough." Calli imagined her girl in elementary school and during her teenage years and hoped she'd be "just cute enough" to not gain attention from what had happened after her birth. The helmet brought these fears to the surface, these motherly worries about the mental, physical, and social well-being of her child, but eventually the helmet became part of Xaida and their family, and eventually the child's calling card, one that would gain her notoriety at church and at Calli's other children's school. Little girls flocked to Xaida at her older brother's school. They ran to ask Calli how Xaida was doing. They doted over her in the school parking lot. When the helmet was removed, people in the community who had looked forward to seeing the little girl's face inside the helmet seemed to miss it. They asked where it had gone. They asked if she would still be protected. They got used to it on her and nearly mourned its absence when it was taken off, proof that a helmet on a baby's head cannot take away the beauty of the baby, proof that the time will pass and that the world will embrace a little one who got off on the wrong foot but was resilient enough to make it through.

Standing at the front of the classroom, Xaida's brother Noah held a poster board up so all of his classmates could see. On the poster board he had taped pictures of Xaida before surgery, right after surgery, and with her helmet on. Instead of bringing something from his room for show-and-tell, something trivial like a signed baseball or a souvenir from Disneyland, he brought in a poster board covered with pictures of his little sister and talked about how when she was born the part of her skull that should have been open was closed. He talked about how doctors went inside of her head and cut out bone. He pointed to her photos with his finger, and told his friends, classmates, and teacher what the helmet did—it prevented the skull from growing one way and made it grow another way. By the end of the talk, hands had shot up to ask him questions about craniosynostosis.

Scarred Detritus

I sat on a bench at Cunningham Park in Joplin, Missouri, and waited to meet Kim, Wes, and their three daughters. At 11:30 on a sunny Saturday morning in early June, kids ran and jumped and swung on trails and playground equipment, including swings. Paths weaved in and out and around the park. Lifeguards trained in the water park at the edge of the road. They pulled dummies out of the water and laid their heads gently on the pavement before leaning over, pumping air with clenched fists into their rubber chests, and blowing air into their rubber lungs. Other guards, standing at the base of the water slides, listened to their coach and watched his hands as they rose into the air and traced the edges of the slides as if he were following the limp body of a child who had hit her head while flailing into the entrance of the chute—then he tapped the young guards on the shoulder and they jumped into the water and rescued the imaginary child. Eighty-degree temperatures, no clouds in the sky, and bubbling energy from kids being watched by their parents who grilled burgers on the outdoor cookers screamed "summer," and smiles and laughter drifted along the waves of grass in the beautiful trimmed, mowed, and designed park.

Almost exactly two years earlier, on May 22, 2011, an F5 tornado tore through Joplin and Cunningham Park. Monstous-sized trees lay on top of cars that lay on top of playground equipment that lay on top of earth shredded like skin sliced with a chain saw. The black and green sky swung its muscular 200 mph one-mile-wide arm across the face of the park and only left shards of destruction on its lawns. Pieces of the medical center next door littered the sand pits and filled the ponds. The park had been thrashed and torn and rendered useless for families. One hundred and sixty-one people lost their lives that evening when the tornado, its wind, and the debris that swung around it and from it ripped through the southwestern Missouri town, and Cunningham

Park sat right at the center of a deep, wicked incision that bled and bled and bled.

While I waited, Jaidyn Clark with her wispy light brown hair sat in the back of her parents' car on the way to meet me. The family—Kim (mom), Wes (dad), the two older daughters and Jaidyn, who was born with her sagittal suture (among others) fused—had spent the morning at a baseball game, in which Wes coached, in their hometown Neosho, Missouri. The game had gone into overtime, so the family was running just a few minutes late. When they pulled their car onto State Highway 49 north toward Joplin, Jaidyn asked a very simple question: "Where are we going?" Although the question seemed like one that any four-year-old child would ask on any given Saturday morning, it wasn't. What Jaidyn meant was, "Are we going back to the hospital?" Her tone said it all with her voice rising upward as she said the word "going?" North on Highway 49 meant so much more to Jaidyn than it did to most people: it meant she might be going to the doctor or, even more common than anyone would want, she might be going back into surgery. The road north scared her. She'd ridden on it too many times for someone so young. She had even developed a phobia about hospitals and doctors, one that gives her nightmares when she is at home and shivers when she comes near the large, sterile structures that had been her home on more nights than she deserved.

"We're just going to the park," Kim told her, but knew in her mind that little Jaidyn didn't completely believe her. Jaidyn had been told that there would be no more surgeries before, having asked the doctor herself, and even though he told her that she was done, the family had loaded up the car, headed north on Highway 49, pulled into Children's Mercy Hospital in Kansas City, and, even though her parents wished that what her doctor had told the little girl before were true, two more surgeries cut into her head after the doctor had so confidently told her that she was done.

When the car pulled into Cunningham Park, when the doors of the family van opened, and when Jaidyn and her sisters burst from the car, Jaidyn smiled a huge smile, and it's my guess that her smile came from the truth—they were going to the park that day and not the hospital. Kim and Wes pulled the girls over to meet me with the imaginary leash that parents have wrapped around their children. After we shook hands and the three young girls said a very polite hello, their feet bounced on the grass and their bodies shook with excitement and energy, but then the girls nicely waited for their parents to let them go play.

"You guys can go play," Kim said to her two older daughters. "Jaidyn, stay with us for a moment." Kim wrapped her arms around the shoulders of her youngest daughter and gave her a comforting only-Mom-can-give kind of squeeze. She ran her hands through Jaidyn's thin, wispy hair, and, like most parents I had met, her fingers instinctively ran gently along the little girl's scar. Jaidyn wanted to break free, to go play, and, most important, to not talk about her head. She was like any other four-year-old—she wanted to run free and break free of the serious world of the adults around her—she wanted to get away from the strange man with his notebook and recorder who wanted to talk about her surgeries and scars and young world. She folded into her mom's arms and kept her shy eyes from meeting mine.

"He had his head opened up and worked on too," Kim said to the girl in her arms who would much rather be sliding down the yellow slide two hundred feet behind her.

"A long time ago," I said, doing my best to become a human and break the ice.

She glanced up at my head for a moment and then glanced away. "Can I go play?" she asked sweetly.

"Of course," Kim said. She let Jaidyn go, and her little legs kicked up dirt and grass as she sprinted toward the sand and playground where her older sisters had been playing for many minutes before her.

* * *

In March 2009 Kim and Jaidyn, three days CVR post-op, sat in their car beneath an overpass on their way home from Children's Mercy Hospital in Kansas City. A tornado swung around and around in the early-spring sky, the green of clouds lingering on ahead of them. They had to pull over beneath the overpass and hope that the tornado would not turn toward them and rip through their lives. It had been a very long ten months for Kim and her daughter, and the tornado just seemed to play an appropriate and not so surprising role in their lives at that time. Kim was scared as they sat beneath the concrete structure that would do very little to protect them if the swirling funnel decided to swing down with a knobby arm and sweep the scarred little girl and mother across the plains like a grand finale to a tough year filled with surgeries, one early on to correct an overgrowth of skin that connected Jaidyn's urethra to her anus, and the life-slaughtering effect when a man leaves a mom alone with three very young girls, one who would need very close attention because her sutures decided to close early and the doctors had to open her up to give her brain some room to grow without bumping into the inner and very possibly her outer skull when the inner one thinned out from the pushing on it from the brain. Kim thought to herself, *This just fits. She's [Jaidyn's] had all these problems and now a tornado has joined in.* The winds did not shift their way, and after five hours in the operating room, three days in the PICU, and a long drive in the way of an angry sky, they made it home, where Kim would have to do it alone.

Jaidyn's story began like most stories of kids born with craniosynostosis. She was born via C-section in 2008 and was handed to her parents for them to hold her. She had a tough start. She began life with the yellowing skin of jaundice wrapped around her little body that struggled to stabilize her sugar level. At her three-month check, her pediatrician saw that something wasn't right. The ridges that formed above young Jaidyn's eyebrows like the edges of two pieces of Play-Doh squeezed together by a child's fingers made it very clear that something was wrong with her head. Her forehead dented inward and there was a prominent ridge above her nose. Then, as the first few months of her life progressed, her head started to take on the shape of a boat with her forehead plunging forward above the eyes and the back of her head darting backward above the base of her neck. The right side of her head, for some reason, however, began to push outward and create a lopsided skull.

The doctor ordered a CT scan. When she walked into the room that day, the doctor gave them the results. They were told, like my parents and many of the other families I have talked to, that Jaidyn was born without soft spots, so in early June of 2009, when Jaidyn was just an infant, the Clarks drove to Children's Mercy Hospital in Kansas City and watched their daughter disappear into the operating room for a full CVR. The doctors sliced away, cutting off her scalp from just above the eyebrows and upward, and like they do in CVRs, they lifted her baby skull off her head and cracked it with a hammer to create pieces so they could mold her scalp and release the brain to grow like it should, using plates and screws that would dissolve over time. Jaidyn was diagnosed with sagittal craniosynostosis and was operated on to repair it. Kim, however, who kept all the medical records from the surgery, scanned the doctor's notes and diagnosis years later. Right there below the diagnosis for sagittal craniosynostosis was another diagnosis: metopic suture partially closed. Jaidyn's doctor never said a word about the metopic suture, leaving Kim to find it on her own and steam about it years later, asking the question that I have asked for years: Why can't they just tell us everything? My parents, still to this day, talk about soft spots but would much rather have known the real terminology. Like the Clarks, they were adults and deserved to know the whole truth. Kim's face, under the sun that day at the park, got redder and redder the more she talked about how the doctors didn't tell her about Jaidyn's metopic suture pre-surgery even if it wouldn't have changed her mother's mind one bit about the operation. She handed her baby girl over to the doctor, and when Kim scanned the medical records and found a more serious and more detailed diagnosis than she was told she, very understandably, felt betrayed.

For the most part, the first surgery was a success, but three years later, in 2012, time after time and night after night Jaidyn woke in the middle of the night screaming and crying with migraines that shook her from her sleep. She was three years old and pain that she couldn't completely explain shot through her head. In the middle of the headaches Kim and Wes had no idea what to do, so they just held her and held her until she calmed down, and then, shortly after the headaches began, they took her back to their pediatrician and on her request back to Mercy Hospital and had Jaidyn's ICP tested—through the use of a spinal tap to avoid the subdural bolt—to find that it was three times as high as a normal child's pressure, and their doctor believed it was because her brain was making contact with her skull, the layers between brain had been stretched too far and thin, and the brain did what it was supposed to do: grow. The pressure in the skull for the young girl should have been anywhere between 10 and 18, but the pressure that pushed and pulled and shrank and expanded in her little skull tested at nearly 36, anywhere between two and three times the amount of pressure that should exist around Jaidyn's brain.

Dr. Staffenberg explained the problems with the presence of ICP and the variables of ICP testing:

> In Paris, they have studied babies with single suture synostosis. They would drill a little hole in the skull, put a pressure monitor in, send them to the ICU, and watch the pressure. About 12 percent of the babies had increased cranial pressure. The problem is, even if you do that, it's not terribly reliable. Pressure varies over a twenty-four-hour period. And in craniosynostosis, one thing we still don't know is that even though a baby may not have signs of increased cranial pressure, when we operate we'll see the bone on either side of the forehead in this area is much thinner than the rest of the bone. And why would that be? It's only because the frontal lobes of the brain are trying to push the forehead out to the side like this. And as it's pushing, the bone is designed, like I said before, to actually be taken on the inner table. And deposited on the outer table. If, that is, if the brain is pushing hard enough, it'll eventually thin out. In babies like this, bone actually becomes like Swiss cheese because the brain is literally pushing through it. There's only a certain amount of bone, so if the brain is pushing against the bone hard enough to thin it out, then there's constant pressure of the brain on the bone; even though there's not increased pressure in the head, that pressure on that part of the brain is back there. And we're not able to measure intellectual performance in babies of that age in any reliable way. We're not able to do that sort of testing. We have heard, anecdotally, parents tell us before and after an operation, "Oh, they blossomed. All of a sudden they're doing these things that they didn't do before," but we have no scientific way of evaluating that, so, you know, increase in cranial pres-

sure is one thing, but I think there is a different kind of pressure that these babies are vulnerable to. Babies that have sagittal synostosis, we'll frequently see during the operation the inner layer of the bone, especially if the back [of the head] is irregular, scalloped, something that we call "thumb printing" or a "copper beaten appearance," and that is the same thing. It's the brain pushing up against the bone. When we look at a normal brain, there's a little bit of space between the skull and the brain, cerebral spinal fluid there and everything else. If the brain is that close to the bone, then that pressure is irritating.

To bring down the ICP, Jaidyn's doctor first prescribed Diamox, a drug typically used to increase spinal fluid to float the brain and keep it away from the skull, therefore reducing the ICP. Then he scheduled a surgery for her for September 2012 to put in expanders to stretch her scalp to reduce the contact between the brain and the skull. They took her away again.

The expanders were placed under her skin and at the back and back top of her head like two thick uninflated balloons beneath a thin sheet of cloth. Her doctor felt that her scalp clung too tightly along the hardness of her skull; therefore, when he looked at his options he felt that there just wasn't enough room for him to do another expansion without the use of expanders to stretch out her scalp.

Her surgeon opened up her previous scar, revealing the dark red dura beneath her skin above her ears, and placed the clear expanders beneath her flap of skin and closed her up again. The expanders come in many different shapes and sizes, and it is the surgeon's choice which to use based on the patient's needs. Once the expanders were placed beneath the skin at the back of her head, the doctor ran the filling tube along her hairline and over her left ear from the back of her head to the front of her head and opened up two small holes, called ports, centered between her ears and her eyes; the ports were made of metal with a rubber lining to protect her skin from the contact with the metal. Saline would be injected into the hole twice a week to fill the expanders and therefore expand the tissue around the bone that needed to be reconstructed. He planned to open her up and do another full CVR to reconstruct the skull, as he felt there was enough deformities throughout her skull that another CVR would be necessary to fully correct her head.

Twice a week, Wes and Kim had to take a butterfly needle, typically used for an IV, full of saline in their hands, hold their daughter still long enough to stick the end of it into her scalp through the little hole in her skin, and hope they did everything right. At the table in the park, Wes rubbed his hands together in contemplative worry, and as if he were back in time and he were aiming his hand toward her head, he mimicked the motion of pulling his index and middle finger toward his stable thumb, the imaginary injector clearly in his hand.

They live in Neosho, Missouri, nearly three hours from Children's Mercy Hospital in Kansas City, so they couldn't make the drive north twice a week to have a specialist inject saline into their daughter's head, so they had to do it themselves, and this tore through Wes.

"The expanders were hardest on me. Out of all the surgeries and everything, the scalp expanders were hardest on me," Wes repeats two or three times before he explains why. Before her second surgery, Jaidyn's doctor wanted to avoid too much pressure on the sutures that would inevitably come from expansion after reconstructive surgery, two months before her second surgery in September of 2012 when she was four years old, so her doctor inserted tissue (scalp) expanders to do a lot of the expansion work before the cranioplasty. When the skin is expanded using a tissue expander the epidermal thickness increases. However, after removal of the expander, the epidermal thickness gradually returns back to normal after four to six weeks. The pilosebaceous elements are well preserved, although they may be compressed on histological examination (tissue regeneration during tissue expansion and choosing an expander).

"I mean, it's my own daughter's head. I'm not a surgeon or a nurse or a doctor," he said. "We had to do this twice a week because we were nowhere close to the hospital."

"We live two hundred miles from the hospital, so they just gave us all that we needed to do it ourselves, and we did it," Kim said.

They hated doing it, putting Jaidyn through that and watching the skin on the back of her head creep and creep outward until her head revealed the shapes of the expanders beneath her skin. Distinct lines in her scalp and skin outlined the expanders beneath them like the creases on the top of rolls created by the rising and falling of the yeast. The front half of her head looked normal, minus the injector hole on the side of her scalp, but the back rose and fell with canyons created by saline injected into the expanders.

"I hated doing that," Wes said. "I mean, it's my own daughter. She hated it, and I hated that she hated it and that I had to do it to her."

Two weeks after their doctor had opened up the fleshy bright red skin of their daughter, he quit his job at Children's Mercy Hospital in Kansas City. A flood of uneasiness and worry and the fear of the unknown came whooshing through their lives again, and the hectic flow of new appointments, a new plastic surgeon, and a new neurosurgeon nearly drowned the family in anticipation.

They met a new doctor at their next appointment who didn't see the value of the expanders and decided to put in a subdural bolt in in early November 2012 to check for ICP. At that point, he planned to address the need for another full CVR or look at other options, leaving the expanders in during that time, predicting that, no matter what, Jaidyn would need to go under the knife again shortly and feeling that there was no need to reopen her CVR scar until he knew what would the best surgery for her to correct the continued awkwardly shaped right side of Jaidyn's head.

After her third surgery to put in the bolt to test for ICP, Kim walked into the recovery room. Jaidyn was awake and very concerned about what she had just gone through. The doctors put her under and then drilled a hole into her skull. Then they inserted a subdural screw into the hole, wrapping it in and inserting it through a membrane to protect the brain and spinal cord (the dura matter that is wrapped around the brain). This allows the doctors to get a subdural reading of the internal cranial pressure, giving the surgeons immediate data about the child's ICP. The little girl had to stay in bed for two days while they checked her ICP. The reading from the subdural bolt came back at the high end of normal, but these tests are less than reliable; however, Jaidyn had been on Diamox for months and therefore there was some hesitancy by all to say that the pressure in her skull had dissipated naturally.

Little Jaidyn, her hair barely half an inch long after her surgery earlier in September, sat up on the hospital bed in her animals-holding-balloons surgical scrubs. Wires surrounded her like an infestation of weeds. From her head a long tube extends outward toward the wall behind her. It is rubber and the wiring that tests her ICP can be seen running along the center of it. A blood-dampened and discolored sponge wraps around the bolt and the tubing at their intersection, and Jaidyn's eyes can only be described as worrisome; they glance to the right and look at Mom or Dad on the side of her bed.

Jaidyn looked up at her mom and with those same concerned eyes spoke. Wires surrounded her. A bolt with rubber tubing shot out of the top of her skill. A monitor was stuck to her chest below her left shoulder.

"Look what they've done to me," she said. Then with her right hand she pointed toward the IV sticking out of her left hand. On such a small hand the IV was big and cumbersome, and the tape needed to secure it left little room for any skin on the top of her hand to peek through, but Jaidyn's mom nearly laughed at what had upset her daughter as a subdural bolt and wires and tubing were attached to the inside of her daughter's head. Doing her best not to hide what was happening to her daughter and doing her best not to sugarcoat the severity of the situation, Kim gently asked Jaidyn to run her hands over her head to feel what was happening up there. Jaidyn ran her hands over her head until she felt the bolt and tubing between her fingers. Then she dropped her hand down again and pointed at the IV on the other hand and repeated, "But look what they've done to me here." Kim laughed.

The ICP results convinced their new surgeon to stray away from the full CVR, so when Jaidyn came back to the hospital a couple weeks later for surgery on November 12, 2012, her new doctor took the expanders out and redid the right side of Jaidyn's skull, as well as a scar revision. Her scar had grown to nearly an inch wide since the expanders were put into place in September, forcing her hair to part along the sharp ridge of her scar line and eliminating the chance of covering up the history of her short life then laid out like a red, fleshy chronological map on her head.

When Jaidyn woke up in the recovery room and her doctor came in to talk with her and her parents, she looked up at him and with the honesty only an innocent child who had gone through so much could ask she said, "Is this my last surgery?"

"Yes, it is," the doctor said to her before he left the room.

"She's so brave. We're so proud of her. She did so good," Kim and Wes say nearly simultaneously as their eyes drift upward and their minds picture their daughter lying in bed for three days with the bolt sticking out of her head.

The promise about no more surgeries would be broken. Later that year, in early December, Jaidyn fell under the knife again, this time to get tubes in her ears, her tonsils removed, and her nose cauterized because she had been prone to too many nosebleeds in too short a time for her doctor's and parents' comfort level.

* * *

Jaidyn spent a lot of time in the hospital in Kansas City during the fall of 2012. Before and after her surgeries and appointments and checkups and blood work, she played with the all the other kids who had to call the hospital home for large chunks of their lives, some of them having to call it home for the rest of their young lives. She played in the playroom with them, saw them in their hospital beds, and talked to them—unlike some of the other children, after her surgery Jaidyn got to go home, and the young girl of only four years of age knew this and understood that although she had a rough beginning of life that consisted of too many trips to the doctor and too many vacations in the hospital, she was blessed.

One morning in the fall of 2012 between Jaidyn's surgeries, Kim drove her daughter and her friend to school. The fall had started to shift into winter.

The warm nights of southern Missouri turned into the chilly reminders that this world keeps turning and that winter was on its way. When the chill covered the windshield of their car and when T-shirts were replaced by sweaters, Jaidyn and her friend, like most children, thought about Christmas.

From the backseat of the car Jaidyn said, "Can we bring presents to the other kids at the hospital?"

Everyone has a chord, and this comment struck Kim's. She talked to Wes. Both of them knew they had to make this happen. They rallied a group of local ladies to push for the toys—new toys and blankets and stuffed animals—and the group brought in nearly fifteen thousand dollars' worth of gifts for the children at the hospital. Beyond that, Jaidyn's school did a stocking stuffer drive that filled twenty-five boxes with stocking stuffers. Wes, being a member of the National Guard, spoke to his military family—his unit—and his military family chipped in quite a bit as well, another family welcoming the little family into their fold. Wes's boss donated a truck and trailer, and the gifts filled the trailer to its edge, and his boss drove the truck two hours north to Kansas City to meet Jaidyn in her wheelchair the day after her new doctor had pulled the skin back off her head, removed her expanders, reconstructed the right side of her skull, and closed her up again.

Jaidyn, in her wheelchair, covered up in a flowered blanket was wheeled out to the truck. Boxes upon boxes of gifts were being hauled out of the truck by her dad, each of them filled to the top with Jaidyn's hope for a better Christmas for her friends. Red, blue, and bright green gift bags lay on top of the boxes, ready to be filled and handed out. And that's exactly what Jaidyn would do.

Wheeling through the hospital, she handed out gifts to kids in bed, to kids in their parents' arms, and to kids in the playroom. She hugged her friends and gave them a "Merry Christmas," all while the incision in her head pulsated up and down.

Earlier that year, she looked around the hospital and saw the rooms around her filled with children who would not be able to make it home for Christmas, so when she talked to her mom and Wes and told them that she wanted to collect toys for all of them and bring them to their rooms so they could all have Christmas too, she was more worried about the other kids than herself, so her parents could not deny her request and took up her cause.

"She has a big heart, this one," Kim says right before her three daughters began to pressure us to get a move on.

We were just about finished in the park that day when Jaidyn and her sisters ran back up the table where their parents and I sat and talked. Jaidyn wanted to swim, but the pool was closed for the lifeguard training. She became squirmy with nervous energy, and I believe she wanted to get away from the guy with the notebook and the microphone who had monopolized her parents during their day at the park.

"Can we go-o-o?" she asked, in the tone that holds on to the last word, "go," like any child her age would ask.

"We're almost done," Kim said to her. She pulled her daughter in to her and gave her another understanding hug.

"Can I go in the pool?" she asked. Her older sisters stood next to her and leaned on the slivery wooden picnic table.

"We didn't bring our suits," Kim said. "And I promise we're almost done."

"I hate that all of this has changed her," Wes says, and Kim nods in agreement. Their eyes fall toward their shy daughter. Her fear of doctors has grown and her symptoms of anxiety have gotten severe enough that she sees a therapist to help her release some of those fears—this couldn't be easier to understand. "It's changed her personality. Since the last grouping of therapy in the fall of 2012, she has become more guarded. She won't say a word when she gets hurt. She knew that the last time she told them she had a headache, it started a whole series of doctors' appointments and surgeries and scars. Every time they have to give her medicine she thinks it has to do with her head and an upcoming surgery. I hate that it has changed her."

The question has to be asked, "Why?" Why so many problems.

Dr. Staffenberg addressed this very bluntly, in a way that other surgeons may take offense to, but it seems to be true to me:

> So what's been the difference? I mean, we're not using new medication, you know. It's not because of the devices that we're using. It's not because, you know, my hands are magical or anything like that; it's really just thinking through all of this and it's very similar to, you know, when we separated conjoined twins where we looked at, you know, the experience around the world, the survival for these operations that was reported in literature.
>
> Just by making sort of these commonsense decisions, you know. It's really just comes down to the doctor thinking about the right way to do this.

Does this mean that Jaidyn's doctors made the wrong decisions? That is not my question to answer, but I know what Kim would tell you if you asked her.

Jaidyn stood by her mom, and Kim finished talking about her daughter's last surgery. Then, as if she had just noticed her mom talking into the microphone, Jaidyn gently wrapped her tiny four-year-old fingers around it. Kim let go of it, and Jaidyn brought it to her mouth. A gentle "hello" stands alone amongst the ruckuses of a busy park on a sunny Saturday afternoon in the park. A gentle "hello" floats above screaming kids, clanging toys, and the clicking medal of swing chains jerking against the swing set hooks. One word echoes in my office as I write this: "Hello."

"Hi," I say back, and I hope that she has a good year.

The family left shortly after her "hello," the immobility too difficult for the young kids to swallow, although they swallowed it very patiently and with great respect. They had parked next to me in the parking lot, and they pulled out before I did, as I took my time to load up my briefcase and prepare for an hour's drive. That day in the park they went south toward Neosha, but soon enough, when they pull out of their driveway and head north on Highway 49, the right side of her scalp still protesting against all of her corrective surgeries and pushing to grow in any shape it wishes to, she asks how far they are going up this road. Her parents will not be able to say that they are heading to the park but will have to tell her that they are going to Kansas City to see the doctors, this time to fill in the holes and reconstruct the bone on the right side of her head, which has since caved in on that side, which had been too extended by the use of the expanders (according to the new doctor).

"She's a tough kid," Kim said right after Jaidyn said, "Hi," into the microphone. "She's a tough kid."

Two years earlier, a tornado swung through Joplin, Missouri, and left a mark that has been mostly cleaned up. The physical remnants of the destruction brought on by the tornado are nearly gone as housing complexes and gyms and memorials have been built over the scarred land, but much deeper scars remain in that community: losses that are no longer just physical. Once a cut is made, even if it heals, the cut never goes away.

The Corridor

The I-5 corridor stretches out from Tacoma to Seattle. Tall evergreens line the road on both sides and shield drivers from the mountains on the east and the water on the west. Thousands upon thousands of cars drive up and down the corridor every day. People start at their homes in the morning. They have their coffee or juice or cigarette to get them going. Each and every one has the stresses of life that weigh us as a species down. Every person thinks about the past and worries about the future. But, for the most part, we meet so few people in our lives. Out of the 6 million people who live in the Seattle area, I only really know a handful of them, and if push came to shove, if something traumatic were to have happened at Lukas's birth, I'm not sure who we would have turned to for longtime support in our community. The Seattle, Tacoma, Everett area stretches from Canada to Olympia, but when you and your family are alone in a hospital delivery room trying to give a little guy a new life none of those cars or those people or their worries matter. When I held my wife's hand and leg and watched her push and thought about my son's fading heartbeat I had never been so present in my entire life, and I have never been so in the present since. I never knew what it was like to be a good father, but right then I found out.

Two years earlier, only thirty-five miles north of where Mary pushed to free Lukas from his nine-month home, Shelby Davidson struggled to deliver her son AJ into this world at Swedish Ballard Hospital. She met me in a little coffee shop in Magnolia, Washington. The shop was great for the interview. Next to the rows of dark-stained wooden tables where hipsters and coffee shop goers and commuters sat and drank their coffees from their large porcelain mugs with their large porcelain handles, big enough handles to conceal a whole hand, there was an indoor playground for AJ to run around, climb, and play in while Shelby and I sipped coffee, pushed through the awkwardness of meeting a complete stranger, and talked about his life and lives of all the families and children she had been involved with since 2009.

My little family and I had recently moved from western Washington to Kansas, and I was not only happy to sit in a nice coffee shop but also feeling a bit nostalgic for the part of the country that we had called home for the previous six years of our lives, the state where Lukas was born, and the laid-back people who lived near the Puget Sound. There is something calming and inviting

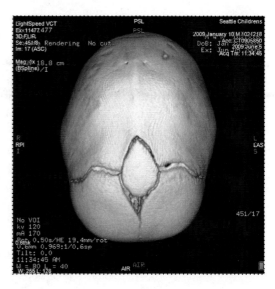

CT scan of closed sagittal suture pre-surgery (courtesy of Shelby Davidson).

about people from the Pacific Northwest that is difficult to explain. They just have a way about them. They seem to smile more gently than others, like there is an ease to it that comes naturally from their mouths and cheeks. They tend to be listeners before they are talkers. This is a generalization, I know, but it is one that I believe in. Last, they are the least judgmental people I have ever met in my travels across this country. I've tried, and have probably failed, to nail down what I mean when I say that people from the Pacific Northwest have a calming air about them, but whatever it was that I failed to nail down, Shelby had it. From the second we started talking, it felt like she was there to put me at ease, the one doing the interview, not the one being interviewed.

AJ was different. "Of course he was," one might say: he had sagittal synostosis. But he was even different from many of the babies who had a fused suture. When he came into this world, his sutures were wide open, free to expand and grow and let the brain shape his head, but as the first few months of his life progressed his sagittal suture closed rapidly and at the edges of the closure a ridge, like many with the same closed suture, began to grow on the top of his head.

"I knew something wasn't right," Shelby said. Like all the mothers interviewed, her intuition played a very large role in her son's diagnosis. The closure was called mild at first, but it got worse and worse as they waited for him to get closer to nine months of age before opening him up and operating, a common practice for her surgeon and one that has proven quite successful for him and his team at Seattle Children's Hospital. Pre-surgery, looking down at AJ from the top, his head was narrow in the front and was shaped like a rectangle had been sanded down around the edges. Above his temples, his head expanded left and right drastically and then narrowed again, this time more evenly, until it became oval like at the back. Imagine, from front to back, a mushroom with a thick base and a narrow head. His 3-D CT scans, taken four months before his surgery, show clean and open sutures on the front and the back of his head and a well-defined anterior fontanel, shaped like a diamond with the lambdoid sutures extending down the sides of his head. Where the sagittal suture should be wide open like a river connecting to lakes, the bone is thick and smooth, the 3-D image of the skull as clear as day and the bone itself like the rounded porcelain of the coffee mugs that day at the coffee shop. While the mugs need no breaks in their clean, smooth edges, AJ's skull needed a big cut right down the middle of it, one that was completely closed up and gone, as if it never existed in his skull.

Through research, I have seen 1 in 1,000 down to 1 in 4,000 children born with, or, as in AJ's case, fused quickly after birth, a syonostosis of the suture that connects the fontanels and runs the nearly the length of the head. There is no controversy about the sagittal suture being the most commonly closed suture, while there is some evidence to suggest that metopic and coronal are catching it in cases diagnosed. There are typically three main ways to release the sagittal suture. Using the CVR as discussed in previous chapters and used to release Wyatt DeVooght's sagittal suture, is very common practice and has been a common practice for more than four decades. The use of the endoscopic procedure, developed by Jimenez and Barone and used in the case of Xaida Rhoades, has become very popular among today's leading surgeons, and then there is the Pi Plasty procedure, developed by Dr. John A. Jane in 1976—many doctors, including Dr. Jane, believe that the Pi procedure does a good job re-creating a more aesthetically pleasing head shape than the previous two— to make a more "rounded contour of the biparietal areas," or in other words, these doctors feel that they create a more naturally rounded curve from the forehead to center of the head, avoiding a squared look at the top of the head, and that will fare better on the cephalic scale by using the Pi technique. The Pi craniectomy has been modified in many different ways since Dr. Jane brought it into the surgical landscape of craniectomies to release the sutures in 1976, coincidentally the year I had my reconstructive surgery to correct my synostosis.

The Pi method gets its name from the Greek letter pi (π). When the strips of skull are excised to release the sagittal suture, the red, exposed dura left without cover of bone resembles the Greek letter π, with the top of the letter facing forward (parallel with the child's forehead) and the legs of the π symbol running front to back above the temporal bones (the side bones above the ears) of the skull and leaving the fused sagittal bone and suture floating in the middle of the π legs. The procedure has become very popular with surgeons hoping to perform a less invasive surgery than the CVR but also provide more surgical shaping than the endoscopic technique and eliminate the post-surgery helmet.

Some people are put on this planet to help others. Some people are put on this planet to give to others. I don't know what Shelby Davidson did before her son AJ was diagnosed with sagittal synostosis after being cleared by the doctors for the first few months of his life, the notes and files and documents confirming that his doctors had done routine checks of his sutures during that time and given an okay during each check, but if she wasn't a helper and giver and a caretaker before this happened I would be surprised. Once AJ and her family had gone through nine months of fear and worry and surgery and recovery, Shelby started to reach out to other moms and dads whose children had been diagnosed with craniosynostosis. First, she started to send care packages to families around the country who were to hand their children off to doctors and go sit in the waiting room for hours and wait. The care packages, the beginning of Cranio Care Bears, provided families with all the essentials they would need for their multiple-day stay in the hospital. She sent one to a woman in Nebraska, who, in turn, paid it forward and sent one to Summer Ehmann, who, in turn, paid it forward and, along with Shelby, started Cranio Care Bears, which, as stated previously, has grown to send packages all over the world and won multiple awards for its generosity. The packages are amazing, and throughout my research for this book I have not met a family who failed to not only receive a package but also appreciate the package immensely when it came in the mail on the day of the surgery, the support that it represented, and the legitimately useful list of toiletries and books and snacks.

But Shelby did not start with the shipping of the packages; more than a year before starting Cranio Care Bears, she opened her life to others. In the early days, at the end of 2009 and before families sought her out through word of mouth and Cranio Care Bears, Shelby contacted them. She reached out to *them* and asked if they needed anything from her, any advice, any answers, or any comfort. Some never got back to her. Some got back to her immediately. And some have never left her life. This kind of giving doesn't end after diagnosis, after surgery, or after recovery. It lives and breathes and pumps the hearts that have been touched by craniosynostosis, or any other major birth defect for that matter, and it is a lifelong investment that Shelby gives whole heartedly every time she contacts a parent or one contacts her. Some ask her to just answer questions through e-mails. Some ask her to sit with them during the surgery. And some ask her to, understandably, stand by them through every doctor's appointment and surgery and in the recovery room. The family aide badge that she wears into the hospital during the surgery is not just one of practicality for that day but also emblematic of what she gives before, during, and long after the young children leave the recovery room.

"Going through all of this, even though I had a very supportive family, I felt lost and alone," Shelby said. "I vowed then and there that I would be there for any family who faced this to help them if they wanted my help."

Within one month post-op for AJ, Shelby sat in the University Village shopping center just outside Seattle Children's Hospital and made good on her promise, her innate desire to help others who had to go through what she went through and was currently going through. She waited for the Colvins, the first family she would meet after AJ's surgery, and the sky did what the sky did in Seattle in November: it lay covered in clouds, and the cold winds from the Puget Sound swept westward across the water and fell onto the city. The Colvins came with a diagnosis from the doctors: craniosynostosis. The family was nervous. The emptying clouds mirrored their eyes. Shelby had AJ with her. He sat in her arms. His scar was still fresh and still shone brightly beneath the lightness of his returning hair. He looked much differently than he did pre-op, and Shelby, while she was able to help the Colvins by forecasting their lives over the next nine months and ease some of their worries by pointing to her son, who was doing so well after surgery, his beautiful smile popping out beneath the clouds of the Pacific Northwest, felt an inner turmoil had begun to rumble and shake, like a dormant vol-

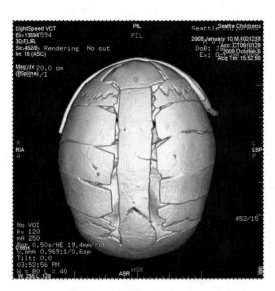

CT scan of modified pi surgery to release sagittal synostosis (courtesy of Shelby Davidson).

cano coming to life, deep down in places she didn't know existed, and her sub-conscious did its best to keep the lid on.

In 2010 during my son's ultrasound in Tacoma, I don't know what I prayed. I don't know if it made any sense. But I prayed hard. My wife, Mary, and I sat in our midwife's office and waited for the ultrasound technician to come in and scan Mary's belly. I didn't say a word to Mary about my worries because I didn't want to voice them—I didn't want to give them credence or fleshiness. I sat quietly, and Mary interpreted this as a disregard of the impor-tance of the moment—we would be seeing our child for the first time through the medical gift of sound waves. Her assumption couldn't have missed the mark more. The severity of the moment had found its way into the marrow of my bones and rang with the pain of worry, anticipation, and foreboding conclusions and, like a the pain of a phantom limb, I could feel the nerves in my skull and count my pulse as it pushed my large forehead vein toward the edge of skin.

Before the ultrasound tech wheeled her machine through the open door of the office Mary tried to hold my hand, but I pulled it away slightly and placed it on my forehead, hoping that it looked like I needed to wipe the sweat off my brow, which was only a half-truth. She gave me an odd look. I'm the affectionate one in the household, the hugger and squeezer, and it wasn't like me to pull my hand away from her generous affection. But before this pull of the hand could turn into anything besides a quizzical look, the tech walked into the room and Mary's attention, rightly so, was no longer pointed at her quiet, sweating husband with his hand on his forehead.

The tech lifted Mary's shirt to expose the slightly rotund belly. Her skin had started to shine from the stretching of her skin, and her belly button had expanded to form the biggest outie I had ever seen, and it was all beautiful and perfect in a way that I could have never dreamed. The tech's hand cupped the ultrasound ball and moved it in circles on the mound of belly in a hunt for mine and Mary's baby. Then he, our son Lukas, appeared on the screen in multiple shades of black and white. He had tucked his legs into his chest and pushed his fisted hands up above his head into the top of the womb, punching at Mary's insides. But his scalp, the one part of the body I searched for, could not be seen. Then my prayers became focused and clear: *Dear Lord. Don't let him be like me.*

"Now there's his little heart," the tech said. She kept the ball on top of his beating chest to record his heart rate. "Good, strong heart rate," she said.

Mary cries over cheesy sitcoms, and up to that point she had not let a tear go. I was surprised, completely surprised, but when the heart pounded on the monitor next to her left ear, tears escaped from her eyes and fell onto her cheeks. She glanced at me and laughed with tearful happiness, but I remained quiet, and when she turned her head back to the screen, without thought I moved my hand from my forehead up past my super-receding hairline and found the edge of my scar and traced it from the top of my forehead to the back of my crown. The bumps beneath the scar rose and fell under my finger-tips like hardened bubbles on pizza crust. The outer edges of the scar riveted against the skin on my skull, and the few strands of hair left on my balding head stood up.

The tech scanned over Lukas's skull and continued on. I yelled at her in my head to stop, to look closer and longer at my son's skull, but she passed on by to check the sex of the baby. She paused for a minute over Lukas's genitalia, and I just wanted her to rewind. Most parents want the tech to pause, to look at their child's genitalia, to hover over the organ, or absence of an organ, that would define their child's life in most every way, but I didn't give a rat's ass if my child was a boy or a girl; I only cared about his skull, and the tech quickly passed it by.

"Everything looks good for your little boy," the tech said to Mary, and then glanced at me momentarily—I looked like a husband who had no interest in what took place that day. I was completely silent throughout and held my hand on my head like I had made a mistake. But finally, after the tech had said she'd seen no problems, I reached and grabbed Mary's hand as she cried and laughed and smiled all at once.

I could not hold Mary's hand in the midwife's office that day because I had assumed the guilt my mom had lived with. I had been begging forgiveness for the slightest chance that I might transfer the gene to Mary's son and the chance that I might put her though my mother's hell.

* * *

Drs. Andrew Wexler and Leslie Cahan, a surgical team based out of LA, had been performing a modified version of the Pi craniectomy, like what was done in AJ's surgery, and chronicling their results for more than fifteen years (beginning in 1998.). With their modified version of the traditional Pi method, they remove the temporal bones and divide it into three horizontal strips instead of three vertical strips, bending the temporal segments and sewing them together to create a bone graph that looks like a venetian blind; this technique is also referred to as the Venetian Blind Technique. They saw very good results from 1998 to 2011, mainly consisting of very rounded biparietal areas of the scalp and high scores on the cephalic index. Most doctors who perform the Pi or modified Pi craniectomy, as in AJ's case, believe the ideal time for surgery is between five and seven months. In this case, "A coronal stealth incision is followed by reflection of the scalps flaps posterior as far as the lambdoid suture and anteriorly to just beyond the coronal suture" (Wexler and Cahan). Then, similar to an old-school strip craniectomy, they use a saw, a very tiny saw that can be held in one hand, to cut around the bone where the sagittal suture should be and remove it. The removed suture is typically a width of three to four centimeters. The Pi leg, the strip of bone between the removed sagittal strip and the to-be-removed temporal bone, is retained, therefore forming the top leg of the Greek letter pi: "A segment of bone measuring 1.5–2 cm is removed from the anterior portion of each Pi leg maintaining adequate bone posterior to the coronal suture to allow for subsequent fixation. Three drill holes are placed at the anterior end of each leg with a complimentary 3 three drill holes placed 1 cm posterior to the coronal suture" (Wexler and Cahan).

From there, like professional tailors of the skull, the doctors thread #25 steel wire through the central drill holes that are threaded with absorbable sutures:

> The wires are tightened, shortening the anteposterior (AP) [the difference between the front and back of what is being measured] diameter and displacing the brain laterally. When optimum AP shortening has occurred, the sutures are tied and the wires removed. On the back table, each temporal bone is cut into three horizontal strips. The strips are shortened to correlate to the foreshortened skull configuration, and a bone bending forceps is used to contour the bone to the shape of the protruding brain. Two drill holes are placed at the superior and inferior aspects of each bone strip to allow for 2–0 absorbable sutures to connect the strips of bone in an articulated fashion like a Venetian blind. The bones are then replaced to the temporal position on the skull and held in position by suturing them to the Pi legs bilaterally. Barrel stave cuts are made in the temporal bone anterior to the Venetian blind to contour the transition between the construction and the coronal suture. The scalp is closed over a closed suction drain and interrupted 4–0 dermal sutures followed by a running skin suture of 4-) plain gut [Wexler].

While this technique is very similar to what AJ had done, and it stays consistent with Dr. Jane's initial construction and methodology from the 1970s and then again in the 1990s, it shows that while the technique is quite common, it, like the CVR and endoscopic methods, is continually changed, modified, and adapted to the circumstance of the child on the operating room table and the advances in the field of cranial facial surgery.

In AJ's case, his doctor used a very similar technique to the Venetian Blind Technique of the modified Pi technique. When they opened AJ up that day, they found that his sagittal suture was no longer a mild to moderate case of synostosis and, as noted before, the area between fontanels was as shiny, solid, and clear as any rounded edge of a porcelain mug except one thousand times stronger. His doctors at Seattle Children's Hospital cut an incision, zigzagged from ear to ear (the most common shape of incisions these days), and pulled his skin backward and forward from the incision to reveal the skull. Then, with their saw, they began the creation of their π, cutting out the skull behind the forehead to create the top of the π, cutting out two slits around the fused sagittal suture to create the legs of the π. From there, they removed his temporal plates, just like in the Venetian Blind Technique, but instead of breaking the temporal bones horizontally, they made the breaks vertically, like the blinds had been flipped sideways—this would give the brain the chance to grow outward without much resistance, with the gaps around the ossified suture and the slits in the bone on the temporal sides. Then they put him back together. To the laymen, it sounds so simple, but it is the furthest thing from simple, as the hands of the surgeons have to cut the bone exactly, bend the bone to shape the child's head precisely, and then put everything back together to create not only a better-functioning skull but also a more rounded biparietal shape, hoping that no one will ever notice that at nine months the young boy would have such a deep-rooted connection to the Greek letter π.

AJ's surgery went as well as any other surgery could have gone. He went in to the operating room with a closed sagittal suture and came out with, as his post-surgery X-rays show, a long strip of bone lying on the top in the center of his skull down where his suture should have been. Two distinct boneless spaces lined each side of the bone like long, thin window panels on the side of the front door of a home. His temporal (side of the head) bones had long slits that fell down the side of his head from the top of his head to above the ears. The long bone in the center of his head, as well as his temporal bones, was attached to the front and back of his skull. They closed him up and stitched his zigzagged scar together, one that looked like the black zigzag on Charlie Brown's shirt, stretching from ear to ear. This reconstructive surgery had a very distinct effect on AJ's skull shape, beginning with what before looked like a bean with one narrow end and one broad end, so when he was taken out of the operating room and placed in Shelby's arms his head was much more rounded, even with the abundance of swelling that pushed at all sides of the skin and created a balloon-like look on his recovery face. Where his forehead once narrowed quickly above his eyes, it now had a very nice, very pleasing to the eye (what most people would call pleasing to the eye) softness to it as it gradually rose roundly toward the top of his head on both sides—its symmetry, with the lines of his cheekbones and the curve of his little jaw, was too great to not notice. The narrowing at the front of his head that looked as if it had been squeezed by two hands was gone and reshaped, like that of his forehead, to a nice, round figure that blended into the back of his skull without a quick outward jutting of bone and skin that branded the boy unmistakably as a child with sagittal synostosis.

In the eyes of the world and in line with societal expectations, AJ looked better—"more normal," as many would say; "cuter," as others might blurt out; "like other children," eyes would confirm. But to Shelby, when the doctor came into the room post-op and placed AJ into her hands, and when she looked down her at puffy, post-surgery son, her bright orange parent/caregiver band strung around her neck and her dark hair tied behind her head, she peered down at his newly rounded head with all of the societal-tagged imperfections wiped away with the precision of a very talented surgeon's hand, she didn't see the boy she had fallen in love with since his birth. It wasn't the swelling or the scar or the absence of hair or even the tube of blood that ran from his head and into a plastic pouch; it was his head, his new head, his "fixed" head, his "normal" head.

Soldiers who come home from a battle and have lost limbs or, more important, lost friends in battle; cops who charge into a room and see their partner shot or themselves take a bullet in the line of duty; firemen who climb ladders, wade through smoke, fall through fire-made-fragile rafters that hang above flames only to lose a child to the tongues of heat. These are the people and the circumstances that we imagine when we imagine victims of post traumatic stress disorder, or PTSD. But these brave people, first and foremost, are not the only people out there who see or experience something that tunnels its way into their minds, into their memories, and into the places in the mind that neurologists can name and point to, but still, to this day, they cannot explain in detail how the brain captures, holds on to, stores, and re-creates images and emotions in the body long after a the traumatic event happens.

It's in Shelby's eyes. She holds her little boy and looks into the camera. There is a blankness, an expressionless void that can't really be explained in words but looks as if she is looking past the camera into a white light that holds her tired eyes open. There were a few tears or even hints of tears that had come and then been wiped away—no redness or swelling from the soft edge of a tissue or veins in the eyes that spread out of the edges and meet in the middle. There is a calmness there, but there is no peace. Her little smile says, *I am here. AJ is with me,* and that is all. Of course, everyone who has been in her chair and held their baby knows that surgery is really only a scary, defined step along the way and that there are mountains, maybe less defined, worrisome steps on the horizon, but her face doesn't show fear either. She seems to just be there, to be awake, and to hold her boy after surgery.

"That wasn't my son," she said. "That wasn't the boy I loved for nine months. He was gone."

The days and the nights came on, and AJ got better. He healed up, he went home, his swelling disappeared, and very shortly after the surgery and the recovery had begun he looked as cute and as "normal" as any other baby. His smile, so big and endearing, his eyes wide with no pressure on them, and his big dimples in his cheeks pointing upward toward the soft, flowing edges of his reconstructed skull. But Shelby had yet to cry. She had now made it through the worrisome five months between diagnosis and surgery, through the long wait in the hospital waiting room, and, finally, through the surgery, the recovery room, and the hard weeks of no sleep and the fear that followed, but she had yet to break down, yet to fill her eyes with red veins, and yet to wipe the tissue across her face to clean away running mascara. She had even begun to meet families, like the Colvins, at shopping centers in North Seattle to help them out for a year before sending out the first care package, to a family in Nebraska. But she had yet to let it all out herself, the interior of the volcano boiling and spurting and rumbling at its core. Like the clouds that sit over Seattle nine months of the year, Shelby had yet to reach the end of that long, dark winter in her life.

If looked at against the seasons of the Pacific Northwest, she was in the late months of the cloudy season. Those are the hardest months. The rest of the world is coming out of winter and reporting sunny days, but the Pacific Northwest hangs on to the cloudy season just long enough to even drive locals a bit crazy. Shelby was in the eighth and ninth month of overcast, and the itch for the sun and the lighter days started to surface not in the subtly lifting clouds but on the waves of lava that pop beneath the crust.

Four months post-op, dizziness came over her, tingles shot through the back of her neck, her limbs became numb, and her heartbeat pounded, pounded, pounded faster and harder against her chest until the anxiety attack finally stopped. She thought it was serious enough to go to the hospital, but with her husband by her side she did not go. She wasn't in any immediate danger until it happened again.

The next swirling sickness of panic consumed her; she was driving with AJ in the backseat. She managed to weave her way through traffic, her heart slamming against her chest and the world swirling around her with dizziness and spins, and pull into a fire station. They called an ambulance. She was taken to the hospital and diagnosed simply with tachycardia, the abnormal speeding up of the heart rate, which can lead to a cardiac arrest, but the doctors blamed it on her morning coffee and released her.

It happened again; she saw her doctor again. He said the same thing. This happened two or three times, but she kept coming back. She felt her symptoms were too severe to brush aside and blame on coffee.

She knew it wasn't the coffee. She'd been through a lot over the last year, like all parents of children with craniosynostosis—worry, diagnosis, worry, surgery, worry, recovery, worry—and, in the back of her mind, something told her that it had affected her. She'd experienced something outside the range of the normal human experience that had taken her out of her normal life and placed her in a bubble of numbness. She had yet to cry, let go, or break down about AJ's surgery and had begun to have panic attacks; the pieces started to fall into place—the traumatic events in her life had led to psychological damage such as PTSD, even though her doctor continued to send her home without help and told her to lay off the good Seattle coffee. PTSD, however, is not uncommon in parents, especially mothers, who have had a child be admitted to or spend time in NICU or PICU, occurring in nearly 1 out of 4 parents—21 to 23 percent experience PTSD after their stay, and these are just the reported incidents, as many parents fail to report because they have been told to just suck it up or that it will all get better or that they should drink less coffee in the morning.

The symptoms of PTSD manifest themselves in parents of children who have been to the PICU in the same ways they do in soldiers, negatively affecting the parents' mental and physical health and their relationships with family, including their children. They can re-experience the phenomena in the form of nightmares, inhibiting their ability to sleep and therefore affecting their mood during the day, they can start to avoid any thoughts or memories of the event or the trauma, and, like Shelby describes, they can be overwhelmed or maybe underwhelmed with a sense of "numbing to general responsiveness," which limits their range of emotion, making it difficult to feel love and happiness, as well as sadness, and they can feel hyperaroused at times, getting jumpy or scared or startled at any time without preparation, something that overcame Shelby driving down the road one afternoon with little AJ in the backseat.

"That wasn't my son," she said. "That wasn't the boy I loved for nine months. He was gone." Something else happened that day in the PICU when AJ came out of surgery. Before the swelling begins, parents I have talked with have repeated over and over again that their children look like they will look when they are healed up post-recovery, post-bandages, and post-swelling. AJ looked completely different than he did before surgery, like a different little kid, and Shelby, without realizing it at the time, fell into mourning. The percentage of PTSD in parents, especially mothers, who have lost children due to illness or trauma rises drastically, and one way of coping with the loss is to avoid any emotion or to be unable to feel emotion associated with the loss. The effects of losing a child, or the perceived loss of a child, as in Shelby's case, are widespread and can alter relationships with family, partners, and even other children, diminishing the chance of emotional connections with those around the affected. What Shelby felt that day and for months after—PTSD symptoms must be present for more than a month to distinguish between them and symptoms of ASD (Acute Stress Disorder)—is not uncommon in mothers of children who have gone into surgery and come out looking like different children.

What needs to be avoided, and wasn't avoided by the medical professional team in Shelby's case, was advice that interferes with support for parents who suffer from PTSD. Too many people give faulty advice in hopes of helping, but all it does is hurt the victims more. Parents should never be told that they will "get over it"; they should never be made to feel weak or like they are exaggerating their symptoms or feelings because another parent dealt with the experience much better; people should listen and avoid trying to relate by discussing their own experiences with the other parents; supporters should never give advice about what works for them if they haven't gone through the same thing; and they should absolutely never tell parents that they were lucky and that it could have been worse. These guidelines to talking with someone who has gone through a traumatic experience are shared among the medical professionals who deal with PTSD victims. They failed to mention, however, that a high coffee diagnosis is legitimate.

On Shelby's fourth visit, her doctor was gone and a new doctor looked at her symptoms more closely than her regular physician, believed that she could be suffering from PTSD, and prescribed her medication to see if it worked. It did. Her symptoms went away.

* * *

Our plane followed the Puget Sound on our descent into Sea-Tac Airport in March 2012. It had been eight months since we'd left for Kansas with the weight of my wife's dad's cancer on our minds and the beginning of new job drifting on my professional horizon. Lukas had slept through entire flight. As soon as we left the Denver airport, his head dropped onto Mary's shoulder and I caressed the hair around his ears and avoided the hair on the top of his head, because every once in a while I could swear I felt a ridge growing on the top of his skull above his sagittal suture, with my continued worry that we missed a diagnosis along the way. Then his eyes fluttered and shut.

Lukas was born in Tacoma, Washington, in April 2011. Mary's labor was intense. She had no "fun time" during labor like our midwife had told us she would have. Our midwife said that once the first contraction came we should hunker down with board games and movies and cuddle time for twenty-four hours because it would be our last twenty-four hours alone before our baby would be a part of our lives—for the rest of our lives. She told us that we could expect mild contractions for half of a day. And during that time we should enjoy ourselves. We did not get that time.

Mary had gone to her weekly pregnancy massage one week before Lukas was due to drop into our world. She lay on the table and let the massage therapist run her hands up and down Mary's belly and thighs and straining hips. Before the massage, I followed her up to the car and carried her purse. I helped her into the front seat. She'd become extremely uncomfortable over the last two days, and bending her knees and falling into the low-level seat of our little Hyundai was not something she wanted to do, so I pushed the seat back for her, put my hands beneath her left arm, and helped her knees lower her body down into the car. She shut the door and then rolled down the window. Dressed in my running clothes, I had already begun to head out onto the streets.

"I put your list on the cabinet," she said. "Can you take care of that today?" "My list" was my labor-preparation bag. The midwife, one month earlier when Mary and I got into the possible labor zone, had told us to put together everything we needed for Lukas's arrival. One month earlier, Mary came downstairs with her labor bag full of everything the midwife told her to pack. It sat at our front door as a reminder of what was to come. My pack, however, existed, but only in the form of a list on the kitchen cabinet. All the essentials were there; they just hadn't been taken from their rightful places in our home and transferred to a bag that I could take them to the hospital in. In the back of my head, I figured I had another week—I expected to have the twenty-four-hour fun labor to pack up. And I was just lazy.

Mary drove away. I ran up the hill, out of our Dash Point neighborhood and up along the streets of Northeast Tacoma. On the way out, the calm waters of the Puget Sound glittered on my right in the rare sunshine of late spring. Houses with big windows and decks moved by on my left, and the world seemed right. The morning was crisp. The sun felt warm on my face. I shed my gloves and breathed in the humid air of the Pacific Northwest. I returned home refreshed—and positive that I had plenty of time to pack up my labor bag, even though Mary's reminder popped in and out of my brain and even though her labor bag sat at the front door ready to be grabbed and carried to the car. Instead of grabbing a pair of underwear, socks, toiletries, and snacks, I grabbed the Play Station 3 remote control and continued my losing streak as the Seattle Mariners.

That's when my phone rang.

"My water broke on the massage table," Mary said. Through the last nine months I had expected a crazy, scared voice, but all I heard was a calm one. She almost giggled when she said it again, revealing how awkward and embarrassed she felt that her water was then being wiped up and the table sanitized by the massage therapist.

"What?" was the only thing that came from my mouth.

"My water broke on the massage table. She said that's never happened to her before. I felt bad for her," Mary said. As always, she was concerned about the massage therapist's embarrassment more than her own. "You have to come get me."

The world spun around me. On the TV screen, my batter took a strike without even taking a swing at the oncoming pitch.

"Where are you?" I said.

"You know where I am. I'm at the massage therapist's office," she said.

"Where is that?" I asked. I could not place it in my mind's map.

"You've taken me here ten times. You know where it is. Honey, I'm sitting outside on the curb because I'm all wet and I didn't want to make any more messes in their office."

"How do I get there?" I asked.

"Honey, you know where it is. Just get in the car and come get me." Her patience waned a bit, and then her voice trailed off to thank her massage therapist, who had brought her some water and a towel.

"Make sure and grab our labor bags," she said before hanging up.

"Okay," I said. "But mine's not packed. Should I stay and pack it?"

"I'm sitting on the curb in a sopping-wet skirt and leggings with a baby coming out of me; what do you think?" she said. Her patience with my idiocy and laziness had finally disappeared when she hung up the phone.

I grabbed her bag on the way out the door and ran up the stairs toward the car.

Somehow, I turned a fifteen-minute drive into a twenty-five-minute drive by missing turn after turn after turn and circling the massage therapy office five times. My mind led me down the same different paths. I thought about my son and his head and what I would have to ask the nurse to make sure that he didn't have what I had, to make sure that he didn't spend his life covering his scar and confessing to friends and girlfriends that he was born with a birth defect like he had done something wrong or, at one time during gestation, checked the box that said: "Yes, I would like a birth defect." I didn't want that for him. I passed another left-hand turn that I was supposed to make to take me closer to my wife, who sat wet and uncomfortable on the curb. Finally, after making mistake after mistake, I pulled into the parking lot. With legs spread and a towel beneath her and a towel draped on top of her, she waved me over. She sat alone with a smile on her face. Then it went away. A contraction hit hard.

"Do we have twenty-four hours of downtime?" I asked.

"No, Kase, my water broke and I'm having serious contractions," she said.

"Well, are they twenty-four-hour downtime contractions? Should we stop on the way home for some cookies and ice cream and movies?" I asked.

"No, Kase. We need to go to the hospital," she said.

"Now?" I asked.

"Yes, now. What is wrong with you?" she asked me. She put her hand around my shoulder, and I dropped my arms beneath her torso and lifted her up off the curb.

"The midwife said—" I said.

"Well, everyone is different," Mary said before another contraction hit her hard enough to stop us in the middle of the parking lot.

We had to stop two more times before we made it to the car. Her contractions went from once every three minutes to once every two minutes by the time I pulled backward into the exit of the ER drop-off and jammed up four cars that were trying to get out of the parking lot the correct way. Another contraction hit, so I put the car in park, ran around to the other side of the car, and pulled my wife out and walked her in to check in before I came back out to a chorus of yells telling me to get the hell out of the way. That was the first mistake I made that day. I held up ten cars like a cork sitting in a bottle of shaken champagne. They yelled and cursed at me. And as dumbfounded and lost as I had been while trying pick Mary up from the massage therapist, I couldn't figure out how to turn my car around and get myself out of the situation. A male nurse had to come out of the ER and do it for me.

The second mistake came after the nurses admitted Mary for good, her contractions too strong and too close together to release her, even though they had signed the paperwork to send us home once or twice.

I chose the curry dish in the cafeteria. There was an option of fried chicken or curry chicken, and I chose curry chicken. Mary sat on her bed and had a major contraction fifteen floors above me while I told the server, "I think I'll take the curry chicken, thank you." Mary had told me to stay downstairs and eat because she didn't want food anywhere near her, so I scarfed down my curry dinner, which was mediocre, in about five minutes' time, my nerves to jangled to enjoy it, and headed back up the elevator to the fifteenth floor to find Mary walking, very slowly, around the circular hallway of the maternity ward. We seemed to be the only family delivering a baby that afternoon—the other rooms that lined the circle were empty and nurses sat in the middle of the circular room and did paperwork while checking on Mary every few minutes. By the time I reached her, she had begun another contraction. She leaned toward the wall, grabbed her belly and the railing, and moaned. She had been given no warm-up, no welcoming contractions, and no game night. Her contractions gripped her and stung deep. I leaned in and placed both her hands on my shoulders like our midwife taught me do at our pre-labor classes. Mary placed her forehead against mine, and I told her that the labor pains would pass soon enough and that I was there and that everything was going to be okay.

When the contraction passed, she responded, "Did you eat curry for dinner? Oh my god, you have to brush your teeth. Curry? Oh my god, Kase. Did they have any other options?" When she finished her questions, another contraction hit; she leaned in toward me again and moaned. Her fingers dug into my shoulder blades, and she mustered enough strength to squeeze out two words: "Curry? Really?"

When her contraction ended, she told me to run and brush my teeth before the next one hit because she couldn't stand the smell of my breath when she leaned in to hold on to me. I turned to run to our room and find the toothbrush, but she grabbed me and told me to help her walk back before I brushed. It took another twenty minutes and the same number of heavy contractions and the forty reminders that I needed to brush my teeth before we made it back.

Knowing another contraction would hit very soon, I searched my bag as quickly as I could—my brother and sister-in-law, visiting from out of town, had packed a bag and brought it to me before the curry incident of 2011—and I threw everything out onto the floor. Before I could find the toothbrush, another contraction hit; Mary yelled for me to lean on and told me to brush my teeth. The gentle request had turned into a forceful order. It took four more contraction and noncontraction intervals for me to brush my teeth. I found the toothbrush, which helped Mary. I covered the brush with toothpaste. Contraction hit. I wet the toothbrush. Another contraction. Then, finally, I was able to scrub the pieces of curry chicken from my teeth and curry paste from my tongue just in time to hold my wife and let her moan on her shoulder and thank me for brushing my teeth. Her labor would last another twelve hours with no break in the contractions, and the only time I left her side was to greet my mom and dad, who once they heard that Mary had gone into labor booked flights and flew to Seattle from Utah. I met them in the waiting room and told them that they were not allowed in the delivery room and that they should go back to their hotel and wait until the baby was born because it would be more comfortable for them that way. They didn't leave until the day became night and the night became early morning, only heading back for a few hours' rest while Mary continued her contractions on through the night and until the final push began at 7:00 a.m. Our baby's heart rate dropped over and over during the night, forcing the nurses and our midwife to rock Mary back and forth to get his heart rate up. Every time I heard the warning beep that alerted the nurses to his dropping heart rate, my heart rate skyrocketed with worry and I held my wife's hand and kissed her forehead and prayed for his little heart to kick into gear and pump a little faster until he was ready to come on out.

Finally, after his heart rate dropped again, they gave Mary the necessary cocktail to speed up the delivery. The time to push had come. I knew the first thing I would see would be my son's skull, and I knew I would be unable to avoid the thought that it might have a fused suture. There were mirrors and handles and words of encouragement in the delivery room, and there was an assistant to the nurse who wouldn't shut up the whole time. She was older and sweet and difficult to understand. She asked the midwife and nurse for updates on their children and their husbands and their jobs and their dogs and their cooking habits and their choice of socks that day and their ... the list went on and on and on. At one point during the two hours of pushing, I saw my wife look at the chatty woman and try to sear through the woman's chest with her eyes.

Sweat fell from Mary's forehead, I held her hand and placed her left leg in the air, and the chatty old lady talked and talked through the pushing. I did everything I could to not tell her to shut her trap, because Lukas, no matter how hard Mary pushed, was not coming out. He wasn't making any progress. The nurse and midwife had started to express their concerns in forms of "hmms" and "hmphs" and "let's try another position." The old woman chatted on and on and on about her dogs and what she had for lunch and how it was supposed to be a nice day for Easter and about everything else in the world I didn't care about.

Then I saw his head. A sliver of his skull, about a centimeter wide, was exposed for a brief moment, and then it was gone again. I got so excited to see my boy for the first time that I told Mary that she was almost there. This was my third mistake of the day. First there was driving in through the out of the ER entrance. Second there was the eating of a curry dish in the middle of a process that required very close proximity with my wife, and third there was this slipup: "You're almost there. I can see him!"

"I am? You can?" A few of her tears had been shed, at that moment, for happiness. She pushed more. It gave her strength to know that I had seen him, although he had disappeared from sight again. To my defense, I had never been in a delivery room before and had no idea how long it could take from first contact, the first vision of his head, to full-on meet and greet with our new child. She pushed for another half of an hour. Lukas's head could be seen a little more, maybe about two centimeters.

"He's practically here," I said when I saw more hair. "And he's got a lot of hair!" This, again, gave her strength, and she pushed and pushed and pushed.

In my defense, I have no idea what labor feels like to a woman and I have never had an epidural, so I had no idea what could and could not be felt in the labor area. I figured she could pinpoint exactly where his head was in the birth canal.

Earlier, when the midwife thought Lukas might just slide on out, she had put up a mirror in front of Mary so she could witness the birth of our son, but because he decided to hang out a little longer before making an appearance Mary, understandably frustrated, asked for the mirror to be taken away.

"I can see a lot of his head!" I yelled.

The chatty nurse chatted and said, "Yes, lots of hair on this little one."

In my defense, the nurse encouraged what was to come also.

Mary, ready to meet our boy and encouraged by our words said, "I want to see him. Can we bring the mirror back?"

So the midwife brought the mirror around in front of Mary, I held on to her hand and left leg, and the chatty woman talked about a nice Indian restaurant on the corner of please shut the hell up. The midwife tilted the two-foot-by-three-foot mirror down so that Mary could see what was happening. Mary raised her head up from her pillow with another push, looked into the mirror, and only saw a two-centimeter sliver of Lukas's head.

"That's it! That's it! You said he was almost all the way out! That's it! The way you were talking it sounded like you could see his whole head! That's it!" She didn't yell at me because she would never let herself yell at me in front of others and this self-control of her temperament followed us to the delivery room, but I wish she would have yelled at me, because the same eyes that had melted the flesh of the chatty woman only moments earlier tore down the center of my skull. I felt as if Mary reopened my sagittal scar with the laser beams that shot from her eyes.

"Take the mirror away," she said to the midwife. "That's it, Kase? That's it? You can no longer give me updates until he is out of me!"

The chatty lady chatted about how this was common and how many women get frustrated, but with one look in her direction Mary finally convinced her it was time to shut her trap. The chatty lady put on sterile gloves and prepped the room for the arrival of our son, I held Mary's leg and hand, and the midwife gave more instructions. For the rest of the time, I stayed pretty quiet, really only giving words of encouragement and holding up legs. Silently, every time I saw more and more of his skull, I thought about craniosynostosis, I got excited and said to myself, *He's almost here*, and I told Mary how good a job she was doing.

Lukas's heartbeat continued to drop and rise. The green line on the monitor bounced up and down in a way that neither the nurse nor the midwife liked. I watched their eyes and their breathing patterns. They tried to be subtle when they looked up at the monitor and gasped in worry, but if I have one personality flaw or gift, it is that I am hyperaware of everything thing that goes on around me. In restaurants, I talk with my wife and listen to every other conversation that goes on around us and debrief Mary when we walk to the car, saying, "Did you hear what that lady and her husband were fighting about?" Or, "I can't believe that kid said that on their first date. He's going down in flames." Or, "That lady has no idea what she is talking about when it comes to football." My wife heard none of it. In my classrooms, my students think I'm really strange because I hear everything they say and comment on every facial expression that they make. If there is an eye roll, I ask why the eye roll. If there is a gasp, I ask why the frustration. When they get together to do group work, I usually plant myself in the desk at the front of the classroom and do my best to stay seated, but all it takes is a whisper from one group member saying, "I'm not quite sure what he wants us to do," to push me out of my desk and over to the group. I'll walk up behind the whisperer and say, "What's your confusion?," or, "I believe I explained what I wanted you to do pretty clearly." Or, if they're not talking about school, I'll chime in on their conversation from the front of the classroom. They hate me for this. I hate me for this. But I can't help it. Like my mom, I am attuned to every facial expression and can't not notice when a nurse and midwife glance toward the beeping monitor and gasp. They glanced and gasped, and I worried. This went on for another hour.

Then Lukas came into the world. Once his little forehead and ears came through, the rest was all downhill. He didn't cry very long but just shook in the coldness outside of the womb where his mom had sung to him and talked to him and rubbed the skin that wrapped around him for the previous nine months. A photo hangs above Lukas's changing table now, nearly two years after his birth. It does not show Mary's face. The top edge of the photo starts below her chin, and the bottom of the photo ends at her waist. All that can be seen is Mary's pregnant belly, covered in a purple shirt and jacket. Her arms fall inward toward her center, and her hands lie gently on the roundness of her motherhood. Between the frame of the glass and the photo, a little sign reads: "I can't wait to meet you." On the days that I pick up Lukas from day care and carry him up to his room to change his diaper, I cup his head in my hand and try to lay him down softly onto his changing table—at two years old this softness thing has become much more difficult—and before his head drops down to the mat he points at the photo of the belly and says, "Mom?," as in, "Where the heck is Mom?" He can't see her face, but somehow he recognizes her there in the photo, and that day in the delivery room my wife got her wish to meet the little guy.

Their first moment together was one of beauty and amazement and biological wonder all wrapped up into one. She held him and felt relief. Happy tears and the biggest smile covered her face. She'd gotten to meet him.

I wish I were so relieved at the time. The nurse cleaned him up, wiping the placental fluids from his body while the midwife talked to Mary. The nurse handed Lukas to the little chatty woman whom Mary had tried to sear and split in half with her eyes during the final stages of pushing.

"Dad," the woman said. "Can you come and hold the baby while I do my tests? Can you come and hold your son?"

I knew what tests she was talking about, the Apgar tests, and I knew what she would be looking for, and I knew that the fear that Lukas would follow in his father's craniosynostosis footsteps might paralyze me, but I had no idea how to comfort a newborn. I'd never been around babies in my life. To be honest, I avoided them because they scared me to death. I used to babysit my nephew while I was in college, but I always invited girls over to help me out with him because I had no idea what to do if the baby cried, if he spit up, if he was gassy. I definitely had no idea what to do with a newborn who just had spent the last twenty-four hours transitioning from the warm, comfortable world of a womb to the cold table lined with a plastic rim and stenciled ruler.

She placed Lukas down onto the table and moved the warming lamp to focus down on him like he was a little rotisserie chicken that needed to remain warm before he was scanned and taken home. He squirmed and cried, and my paralysis kicked in. Mary looked over at us from the delivery bed, her neck craning and twisting to see what was happening to her boy. He cried louder and louder after he left Mary's arms and was placed onto the table.

"Dad?" the chatty assistant said. Her voice stretched out the word "Dad" to sound like "Da-a-ad?" and to mean, "Can you help me calm and hold your son please?"

I placed one hand behind his head and wrapped the other around his torso. His ribs moved up and down beneath the palm of my hand and fingers while the assistant stuck her fingers in his mouth, through his tiny butt cheeks, and between his toes and fingers. She listened to his heart and his lungs and praised his loud cries, saying that the crying was a good thing. She quickly rubbed her hands over his scalp but moved on way too quickly for my satisfaction.

"Did you check his head?" I asked in a tone that is really rare for me: pushy.

"Yes," she said. Then she moved on to scan his skin for any blemishes.

"Can you check it again?" I asked: pushy. Mary's head popped up again from the delivery bed and she told me that it was okay, that the doctor would look at it soon enough. The assistant wrote down all of Lukas's Apgar scores, said that there were a few things they wanted to check again in a few hours, and then handed him back to me, and I handed him back to Mary. Her eyes grew wide, we snapped our first photo of us and Lukas together as a family, and we started a new life together.

My worries did not disappear that day. I would worry every time our pediatrician checked Lukas over. I would ask Mary to ask the doctor to check his head anytime I couldn't be in the office to witness our wonderful pediatrician's examination of his skull. Craniosynostosis can bare its ugliness months after the baby is born, and I knew it.

In photos, Shelby stands at bedsides with a smile. Stunned, tired parents stand next to her and use the bed rails to prop them up. Their hair is disheveled and their eyes are swollen. Their child lies on the bed, hooked up to tube and IVs and asleep in the wonderland of anesthetic sleep. In some photos there are no fathers, only a mother alone with her child splayed out in front of her and Shelby with a hand on her shoulder. The young mother looks at the camera with a smile. Sure, her eyes are puffy and the draining power of worry and no sleep is splashed across her face in the form of the gauntness that comes from continued rubbing of the face with the hands and the dropping down of the head between the knees, but there is a security there too. The young mother leans forward and looks into the camera like a stranded survivor who has made it out from the desert with the help of a lone Samaritan behind her who wears a cotton sweater and a reassuring smile.

The Howards', Charlie's parents', eyes lit up when I asked if they knew Ms. Davidson. Why I used the stilted "Ms. Davidson" I have no idea, but they corrected me quickly and kindly, "You mean Shelby?"

I lost my formal tone immediately. "Yes, Shelby," I said.

"She was amazing," Robyn said, and Tommy, chasing around their boy, chimed in right away, "Without her, this would have a been a lot harder."

We had yet to really start talking when I visited their home the day after I met Shelby in the coffee shop, stuck in that awkward *I'm this random guy coming into your house to talk about your baby* moment, but talking about someone who had helped them through one of the hardest times in their lives really broke down those barriers that always needed to be broken down.

"She did things and knew things that we never would have," Robyn said. She glanced around the room and placed her hand on the arm of the couch and stared out into the ethereal cloud of memory that seems to sit across the room whenever someone needs to latch on to a memory during a time when their body was strictly on survival mode and not let's-make-memory mode, just going through those day-to-day motions, just shuffling through hospital paperwork motions, just living life until their baby got out of surgery safely motions—all of which every single parent has discussed in detail.

"First, she asked so many questions about Charlie that we would have never even thought to ask. She asked questions that we didn't even know needed asking. She met us first at one of our consultations with the doctor. We really didn't know what was going to happen, but she walked us through all the surgical procedures and then, literally, walked us through the hospital and gave us a tour of where we would go into surgery, where we would wait, and who we needed to talk to. At one point, we needed something answered and one nurse couldn't answer, so Shelby took off to another floor, found the person who could answer it, and came back with what we needed. We were so grateful to have her around." Shelby, as with many other parents, offered to help out the Howards at any time during their journey, and, like many other parents, they accepted. They are still friends with Shelby to this day.

I drift a bit back to the midwife's office, to my intense worry about Lukas born with fused sutures and the moments right after his birth when I should have been thinking about the long night that Mary had just had, about my parents, who waited in the room of a local hotel, about what Mary and I would do when we took that little baby home and all the fears I should have as a father, like changing diapers and getting no sleep, but all I could think about was the fibrous joints between the plates in Lukas's head. As I write this, Lukas is twenty-seven months old and, knowing what I know now and having talked to families whose children just went into surgery at five years old, I often run my hands over Luke's head, letting the tips of my fingers trace his skull like reading braille, and feel for any type of abnormal ridge; sometimes his hair binds together and forms a ridge along the sagittal suture and a rush of adrenaline and fear sends tingles through my arms and legs and a burst of breathlessness into my lungs until I clear the ridge of hair away and settle myself down and kiss every inch of his head before he pulls away from his overly affectionate father.

But that day sitting on the Howards' couch, I watched the two of them think back to their time before, during, and after surgery and their faces lit up when they talked about the support they got from Cranio Care Bears, mothers on Facebook, and, most memorably and important, Shelby. It wasn't just her hand-holding. They are a strong couple, which was obvious from sitting with them, and there's a lot of love in that house, but it was more about her knowledge of the procedures, the system, and the little things they would never think to ask about or expect to encounter: the paperwork, the information the doctors forget to tell you, what to expect the morning of surgery, and, one that digs deep into the heart of every cranio parent, what their child will look like when they come out of surgery and don't look like the baby the parents loved pre-surgery and how to deal with it—even if it's just knowing it will be hard, that everyone experiences something and that everyone will deal with it differently and that different way of dealing with the trauma is okay.

*　*　*

The coffee was done that morning I met Shelby in Magnolia. The interview was over. I followed Shelby and AJ out of the coffee shop and shouted another thank-you to them for meeting me.

"Anytime, and if you need anything else from me, let me know," she said back to me not only with the nonchalance of someone who has said this to so many in the past but also with the ease of someone who fulfills that promise. I turned the corner and walked up the quaint Magnolia Street and got into the rental car, and although Lukas was not born with craniosynostosis, a feeling of peace came over me because right then I knew that if he were born with it, we would have had a friend to help us along the way.

The Great Salt Lake

The opaque gray air filled the Salt Lake Valley like smoke in an old pub. In Utah no one ever talks about the thick smog that sits on the city throughout the winter, in this most recently named seventh-worst city in the country for air quality by the American Lung Association. Instead they talk about the inversion, cool air trapped beneath a warm-air cap that leads to a major reduction in circulation, and in Salt Lake City's case it leads to trapped pollution in the Salt Lake Valley that has been known to sit and rot the air and the lungs of nearly 2 million people for weeks at a time. If you say the word "smog" around many (most) Utahans, they will quickly correct you with the word "inversion" or blame California for the bad air that hovers over them and invades their lungs. A quick drive past the refineries that line the mountains of the Wasatch Front and I-15, as they exhale dirty air into the atmosphere, should distinguish the inversion or California argument, but most legislatures tend to ignore the obvious.

I wouldn't take so much offense to the smog that blocks out the view of the city from thirty thousand feet if the Wasatch Front wasn't, and always will be, my home, and the smog over the last thirty years has gotten worse and worse. It has leaked from the immediately adjacent hills that surround the refineries out over my childhood home in Ogden, thirty miles north of Salt Lake City and south beyond the Provo valley—the purple Rocky Mountain basins blanked out by our own needs. I'm not a crazy environmentalist, nor is this book about the environment, but as the plane dropped down through the smog and into the Salt Lake City airport I felt as if I had begun to mourn the death of an old friend, one suffocated by his own decisions.

One week after I met with Dr. Staffenberg in New York City, my mom and I sat with coffee in our hands, my twenty-one-month-old son playing with his choo-choo on the floor in front of us. We looked out onto the South Ogden

Valley. The inversion covered the ground. My childhood home lay beneath it at the mouth of Weber Canyon, but we couldn't see it. Down there, beneath the smog, the five homes where I grew up, sat my birth home. That was where my parents lived when my mom went into labor, when they were told I was born without a soft spot, and where they took me when I got released from the hospital. The smog sat over it, and like inversion had taken hold of the house, our conversation had been blanketed too.

Earlier that week, I made the mistake of telling her what Dr. Staffenberg had said, without explaining all the necessary caveats that made the percentile less daunting, "You were one of the successful fifteen percent then," I told her as if it were just matter-of-fact. I had been trying to keep her from telling her story, although I had heard it piece by piece for the last thirty years of my life. Pieces were all she could ever give. The memory ate her up too much, tore her down as if she were that twenty-seven-year-old woman who cried outside the doors of the operating room when they took me away. "We'll get there, Mom, at the end of all the research and interviews. We'll get there." We had agreed when I started the book that wine would be involved in the telling of her story and that we would wait until the end of the research to not bias any of my findings. I knew that it ate her up to even think about it, let alone talk about it, but that morning, over coffee, with her grandson playing in front of us, a reason to keep smiles on our faces no matter what, she couldn't help herself from clearing something up.

"I would have never gone ahead with it if I knew there was only fifteen percent chance of success, Kasey," she said. Still hazy in the morning, I was caught off guard. "I would have never risked your life. You were a beautiful baby before the surgery. We loved you so much. I would have never have risked it. The doctor told us there was no reason to worry." In my mind, I have never thought that my parents would have made a decision to hurt me. I knew already what she was telling me.

"I know, Mom. Of course I know," I told her. The smell of coffee weaved through the room. Lukas hooted and howled with his choo-choo. My mom's face dropped down to her cup. She put her lips on the edge of the rim and whispered, again, that she would have never have risked it. Another piece of the puzzle was revealed, and it was tough for her to get it out. Two weeks later, she called and told me about how she broke down at lunch with a friend when she explained the premise of my research to her. After that phone call, I offered to keep her out of the book if it was so hard on her.

"You need to finish what you started, sweetie. I'll be fine," she said. And just like that, she sacrificed herself for me, again. The long conversation awaited us.

PART SEVEN: THE MOTHER, THE ADVOCATE AND THE WORD "COSMETIC"

The Dream

Last night I dreamed of surgery—after thirty-seven years, I had to have another surgery to fix my craniosynostosis. In the dream, my doctor was a burly man. He looked more like a lumberjack than a surgeon. His shoulders were as broad as an ox and his eyes were deep blue. His chin was so angular and strong that a line could be drawn on the exact edge of his cheekbones. His blond hair was thick and full and showed no signs of thinning. In a flannel shirt he stood and told me that I would need two more surgeries to fix what had developed along the line of where my sagittal suture was supposed to be. Jutting ridges like the Rocky Mountains I grew up beneath stuck up above my sagittal suture line like a Mohawk made of bone. Then, at the end of the bone Mohawk, a hole had developed at the back of my head.

I was scared.

His partner, I'm guessing another surgeon, was just as big and strong and handsome as the first doctor, except his hair was dark and thick instead of blond and thick. These two men stood over me and talked to me while the anesthesia worked its way into my bloodstream. The blond surgeon handed me one of my son's toys to squeeze just in case I got nervous.

Then, still in a dream, I woke up. I was standing in front of a mirror. They had shaved the little hair I had that covered up the scar. I was nearly bald before the surgery and even closer to baldness when it ended. My scar gleamed a bright red in the mirror and had become longer on both ends, traveling, now, from the top of the space between my eyebrows to the base of my neck.

The doctors stood behind me and said, "Our hands were tied. That is why your scar is so long." I could see the both of them hold their hands in the air behind me. Both sets of fingers shook, almost like in a cartoon where visible lines showed movement between them.

"We weren't able to close the hole," the blond, strong doctor said. "We'll have to go back in again."

I was scared again. I stood in front of the mirror and looked at my scar. It sank into my head as if being sucked downward, and the men behind me, perfect in the eyes of society, disappeared into the darkness. And as dreams go, two minutes later the three of us stood on a hillside and watched a parked car get broken into. The doctors ran to the car, grabbed the vandals, and beat them to the ground. All I could do was stand and watch the men tackle and hold down the thieves.

The doctors came back to me, and, again, they held out their hands to show me how shaky they were.

"We'll have to postpone your surgery," they said.

I woke up next to my wife in bed, dug my head into my pillow, and assured myself that I didn't have to have another surgery. The dream was vivid and real and scary and weird. I wondered why the men were tall and strong with full heads of hair, the exact opposite of who I am. I pictured the Mohawk of bone and the hole in the back of the head and rubbed my hand across my head. But in the end, when I woke up next to my wife, I was able to say that it was just a dream and that there was no ridge or hole and that I was fine.

No Montage

Ella Darnell lay on the couch in the family room of her home in Salt Lake City, Utah. It is early January, and a snowstorm lasting a week has plummeted and covered Salt Lake City and the Wasatch Front. Winter is in full swing in the valley beneath the Rockies that shoot upward to the sky. Their ridges and peaks and slants and hard, sharp rocks tell the history of this earth. Once, long ago, gaps in the earth's crust fell across the land beneath Lake Bonneville and the land was flat. The mountains that look down on the Darnell household, unlike many other mountain ranges, very clearly showed the multitude of catastrophic earthquakes that shook the ground and pushed the rock upward out of the gaps between the massive plates that floated to the east and to the west of the fault line. The scars of the earth jetted up and were left in one layer on the mountainside. Beneath that layer, the rocks lay horizontal to the ground and were darker than the ones above or beneath them. Another layer. Another layer. And another layer. The layers of time scar the earth on one hand but make it beautiful on the other, all telling the history of what happens when the earth is opened up and opened up time after time. The remnants of massive cuts, while beautiful, cannot be covered up or ignored.

Ella, four years old, lay on the couch in her family room. She is covered up with a soft blanket that runs from her shoulders to her feet. Her bouncy curly brown hair pokes out above the blanket above her eyes. Marlin and Dory bounce around the screen, Nemo climbs through the filter in the tank, and the Seagulls shout, "Mine, mine, mine!," but Ella really isn't watching. She is trying to go to sleep. She tosses and turns, digs her head into the couch cushions, and rubs her feet together in multiple thrashing attempts to get comfortable.

Her dad walks over to the couch and sits down on its edge, giving his daughter enough room to continue wiggling. He places his hand on her shoulder, rubs it with a circular and comforting caress, and asks, "Do you want to try going to your room and going to sleep?"

Ella turns away from him and whispers, "No."

"Are you sure?" her dad asks.

"Yes," she whispers before popping her head up to act like she is engrossed in the actions of the fish that talk and swim on the TV in front of her.

"Okay," he says. He continues to rub her shoulder, doing his best to settle her into sleep on the couch. She continues to toss and turn until the movie ends. The nightly dose of melatonin, suggested by her pediatrician, begins to kick in. The softness of sleep begins to take over and from the bottom of the couch her feet stop rubbing together, her torso stops twisting, her hair stops bobbing, and her eyes close. Her mom or dad will carry her to bed when they head off to sleep.

Ella slept well until her first surgery. The Darnells had a nice routine until they handed her over to the doctors to help reshape a skull for the first time at two years old. The first pre-operative diagnosis was enlarged parietal foramina, windows to the brain, and pansynostosis, closure of multiple sutures of the skull, and the first post-operative diagnosis confirmed that all of the

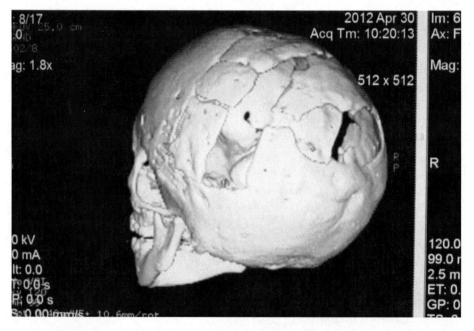

CT scan showing golf-ball-size holes in the back of Ella's skull (courtesy of Laurie Darnell).

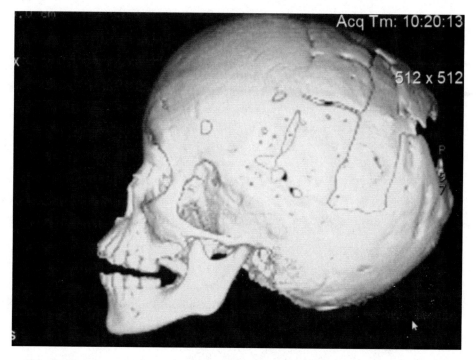

Acq Tm: 10:20:13

512 x 512

CT scan showing golf-ball-size holes in the back of Ella's skull (courtesy of Laurie Darnell).

sutures in Ella's skull had closed. While parents of children with craniosynostosis want soft spots, parietal foramina places large soft spots in areas of the skull that they don't belong. On the back of Ella's skull two large soft spots, the size of golf balls, sat open and squishy. These areas should have been covered in hard, dense skull, which should have been there to protect the brain and growth of the brain, but instead, like two open entryways to the brain, the holes sat agape. Doctors wanted to give them time to close up on their own, give the skull six or eight months to do what it should do, but with the front sutures closed and with the skull distributed and hardened in places that it shouldn't be, Ella didn't have the necessary mass to fill in the holes.

"No one acted on this for two years. The sockets in the back of her skull never closed. Then, the pansynostosis. No doctors acted. Even though we knew they needed to act. Then, at two and a half years old with the holes in the back of her head wide open and all the sutures in her skull completely closed, surgery was urgent," Laurie said. The anger in her squeezes her eyes closed and her hands tense up, grasping at each other like two small animals fighting for territory. In Ella's case, unlike many of the other cases of craniosynostosis, the synostosis may have been caused by the doctors' not correcting her parietal foramina, as the failure to correct the foramina may have directly caused the craniosynostosis—without the ability to watch the skull form, it's only speculation, but Laurie, a pediatric pharmacist who works daily with surgeons and children pre- and post-surgery, feels, "The original defects in her skull may have caused the craniosynostosis, because the sutures likely closed because there was no pressure from the brain to stay open and grow because the pressure was pushing out the back of her head! We may have had a different clinical picture if her skull had been closed earlier." No matter what, no matter the cause, whether there was medical oversight or not, the day for surgery one came, and it was urgent. Laurie and Joe pushed and pushed their doctors to keep looking at her daughter, to make them touch the two open eye sockets on the back of her head and the hard rock that formed the front of her head until the urgency became real enough for the doctors too.

With Ella, with all that had happened to her head in the first two and half years, the back of her skull never completely forming and the front of her skull hardening like cement years before it should, there was no option for endoscopic surgery. Ella's doctors would need to perform a full CVR to release her sutures and fill the gaps in the back of her skull by pulling the entire skull off from the brow to just above her neckline, cutting and breaking it into pieces and then piecing it back together. The day of surgery they laid her in a supine position so they could have full access to her skull. Once they filled her with antibiotics and anesthesia, they placed her in a modified prone position, her little body held tight by chest rolls and beanbags to give the surgeons the best access to her cranium. Their goal was obvious: release the sutures and fill the holes. While this may seem simple and while the doctors used the terminology, taken from her medical records, "Plan today will be to advance the orbits, widen the cranial vault, lengthen the cranial vault to give the brain more room to grow and close the defects," they really just meant release the sutures, structure the skull to make it large enough for brain growth, and fill in the skull with bone substitute mix with any skull that can be taken from the bony plates at the front of the head. As with all CVRs, her head was shaved, the cuts were made with precision tools, and the skull was removed, and in Ella's case the bone was broken up and then put back together to fix the holes in the back of her head with a Plexar substance and bone.

Ella's body immediately began to fight the foreign substances that were used to fill her skull and sew her up. It fought the stitches, it fought the Plexar, and it fought the hardening and growing while Laurie and Joe kept taking her back to the doctor. Abscesses grew along stitching lines, and while antibiotics were prescribed, they did no good at all. The wounds continued to bleed, to release puss, and to, ultimately, get bigger when they should have been getting smaller, turning from bright red to pink, and fading away beneath the regrowth of Ella's curly brown hair.

Two months after her first surgery, Ella again walked with her parents into the hospital, waved good-bye to them, and woke up under the lights of the recovery room in the cold sterile sheets surrounded by tubes and bars and roaming staff. The surgeons went in to clean things up. They swabbed and excised and debrided any scabbing, excess cement from the previous surgery that hadn't settled, and any plates that had not found a home in Ella's head and noted that the cement in her head was very loose in many areas, but they cleaned her up inside and stitched her up again. The doctors assumed that it was a stitch abscess that led to the infection of the plates that were removed, and everything that had been touched by the infection and subsequently pulled out of Ella's head was sent for a culture. Then she was sent home again.

On July 31, 2011, a hot Sunday morning in the Salt Lake Valley, Laurie broke down and, in a way that many do, she wrote to do her best and to do her own excision of the way the world had come back to take a few more punches at her little Ella:

> I'm having a really hard time posting this. I've been emailing my family because it's just too hard to talk about. I'm often asked, "How do you handle it all?" Right now I'm not ... I'm completely breaking. Wednesday morning Ella and I were doing a puzzle and I felt the back of her head. It was soft and squishy ... her poor little head felt the way it used to feel. A few weeks ago this was solid hard BONE and now it's back to mush! I completely lost it! We'd just been to the ER (where we saw 2 doctors) and to her surgeon's office and just had a head CT. Where do I even go next? I called Joe, who was on the ground in Atlanta before his very stressful trip to Mexico. He suggested I call her pediatrician, who has always been our best advocate.
>
> We were the first appointment of the day. After analyzing the situation and spending 45 minutes with us, he called radiology to re-look at the CT describing what he felt. He came back in the room and after seeing his face I just started crying!
>
> The worst possible news: She's resorbing the bone substance. Her brain is no longer covered by solid hard protective bone. We are back to square one! Everyone was so focused on the bump on her forehead.
>
> I made myself so sick that I had to leave work for a while to just get it together.
>
> Why is this happening? How do I keep my very active child safe? Is her challenging behavior a regular 2 year old or is she in pain or just feeling crappy? How do we make the best decision for our precious pumpkin? Why does she have to have every possible complication and the worst case of everything?

I'm struggling. This is the hardest thing I've ever done. We've been through so much and now we have to start all over!

The current plan: We have an appointment Tuesday morning with our surgeon and an appointment in the afternoon with a 2nd opinion. She's in her helmet almost all the time to keep her brain safe.

Ella is happy and does not say she is in pain. I'm putting one foot in front of the other and taking it one decision at a time and one day at a time. I'm focusing on the fact that I have a happy, smart child who I just have to keep that way!

Prayers for Ella to remain safe from brain damage and for Joe and me to collect all the information, ask the best questions, and make the best decisions.

The anguish in her writing, the fear of what was to come, lingers on the Web page. All of the work that the surgeons did during Ella's first and second surgery had backfired. The cement and filler and Ella's bone created a devastating combination of substances that didn't just break down the integrity of the cement, keeping it viscous and keeping it from molding tight and holding, but like a parasite it clawed its way into Ella's healthy bony skull that surrounded it and devoured it too, leaving two large holes, just like the ones that were there when she was born, in the back of her head, two large holes of "mush" that had to be protected, had to be filled, and had to sit on Laurie's and Joe's own minds until it happened.

He suggested I call her pediatrician, who has always been our best advocate.... Joe and me to collect all the information, ask the best questions, and make the best decisions.

These words hang out in her writing like bobbing buoys in a rough surf. Joe and Laurie clung to the only constants they could trust: their pediatrician and their unshaken commitment to doing the best thing for their daughter no matter what it took.

The next day, Laurie sat little Ella, almost three years old, down and told her that she would have to have surgery again. The family had taken a surgery class before her last time under the knife, so Ella dug through her stuff and pulled out a surgical mask, a surgical cap, and some tubing. Then she pulled out her patient: Elmo. In a polka-dotted dress and surgical gear, she laid Elmo down, checked his heart rate, and talked to him while she stuffed the tubing under his arm. Then she patted him until he fell asleep. Laurie had wondered if Ella knew what was coming when she brought up surgery that morning after three doctors had confirmed that all of the bony substance, including Ella's natural bone that had been infected and softened by the infection, would have to come out to keep her safe.

Ella had been in a helmet since her second surgery. The doctors wanted to keep the high-energy little girl from falling and injuring her skull and every-thing inside of it. Laurie made a commitment to herself after finding out that the back of Ella's head had gone soft and on the morning of her surgery con-sultation made a list of eighteen questions for the doctors to answer, psyched herself up to ask every single one of them, and when she walked out the door on her way to the car and the appointment said to herself, *These doctors better be ready for a Mom on a mission to get the information to make the best decisions for her precious little one! I feel prepared and I think I'm emotionally ready for a big day of information collection!* And she got her answers that morning.

Within two weeks of Laurie's running her hands through Ella's hair and finding the softness that lay beneath, Ella went back into surgery. It was rela-tively quick and went well. The doctor went in and excised all the material that he could and believed there was no more of the infection that had spread its tentacles through her skull and seized what it could before placing it in its gaping mouth like an octopus devouring a hard clam and spitting it out again.

Ella had it rough that night and lay in her mom's arms as they watched *Tangled* on TV until Ella fell asleep. Her blood pressure rose and fell, and she, as could be expected, felt very uncomfortable and only asked to be held. The world slowed for the night as Laurie held her daughter in her arms and watched ups and downs of the heart machine as it beeped behind them in the hospital room. Before the surgery, Ella was her funny, smart self. She asked silly ques-tions and pulled Tigger around in the wagon the anesthesiologist would even-tually put Ella in to wheel her back to the operating room. He asked her if she wanted to get on the bed and she said, "No, I'll stay in the wagon." He let her and offered her a blanket so her feet wouldn't be cold. She asked for socks (even though she kept taking them off).

"I don't have any socks," he said.

"My mommy has socks."

He told Ella it was the blanket or nothing and then he said they had to do the mask and she agreed as long as she could do it herself. He let her do it. He let her go under while she lay in her wagon. He was a sweet man. It's these moments, the ones when a three-year-old child knows what is about to happen to her, that give the biggest kick in the gut. Many craniosynosostis children don't know what will happen to them when their parents, with deeply sad-dened hearts, hand them over to the doctors, but the older children who remember their earlier surgeries carry the fear, the anxiety, and the pain along with their mom and dad like remnants from a meteoroid that breaks up in the Earth's atmosphere and burns until it is a solid mass of blackness that sticks into the Earth's crust. Their pain, their memory, eventually may be small, but it is there, and it is real, and it is stuck.

The holes in the back of her head could not stay open. She could not live her life with a protective helmet and no skull beneath it. There would have to be another surgery to fix it. Ella's surgeon, whom she had been with for more than a year and for three major surgeries, suggested two more invasive surgeries to solidify the skull on the back of her head. First he wanted to put in a plastic plate that would protect the brain from injury and solidify the skull. Then he wanted to wait until she was five years old, when all of her bone would be thick enough so he could split the bone like an Oreo cookie and use both pieces to fill the holes without the chance of it wafering. With this approach, there would be a chance of infection and there might be a need to continually go in and readjust the plate, meaning there would even be more surgeries.

Their minds walked through the ins and outs of surgery, the dos and don'ts of pre-op, and the precautions, sleepless nights, and struggles with anesthesia that, like the scavengers that coast along the backs of sharks in rough ocean waters, accompany a trip to the OR. Ella had five surgeries in the previous year, and three of them opened up her skull, knifed through her dura, and skitted along the edges of her delicate brain.

Three-year-olds are active. They love to climb trees and hang from bars and swing from ropes into ponds. They have no fear of injury or death or blood and every three-year-old does their best to put their life on the line every single day and that's normal, but they rarely actually do something that could kill them, that could injure their brain, or that could impact their mental, emotional, developmental, or physical health for the rest of their lives. Ella was an active child from the beginning, with a high-voltage amp that shot waves of electricity through her veins. When she was almost three years old, and Laurie ran her hands along the mushy substance on the back of her daughter's skull that should have been solid bone she was crushed. Ella had worn a helmet for a large portion of her life. Even though she zoomed with energy, she was constantly watched and hounded and protected. Her parents, her grandparents, her day-care provider, and sitters loomed over her like prison guards making sure she did nothing that could cause trauma to her underprotected head.

With this fear of at least another two invasive surgeries and the wait until a minimum of five years of age to complete the cycle of surgeries, the idea of a second opinion wiggled its way into the psyches of Laurie and Joe, mainly because they didn't want to hold Ella back from her childhood and the romping and gallivanting and slamming into life that they had already restricted. At first, they felt guilty about their wanting of another opinion. Ella's surgeon had been with them for years, he met them in the hallways to check her out between appointments, he gave Ella open and unabashed hugs when she asked for them, and Ella adored him. He was a nice man who cared about Ella. After the guilt of leaving him came, the uncertainty and self-questioning followed; the Darnells had been with one of the best surgeons in the area for the last two years. Laurie asked herself, *Would a second opinion around here mean we were getting an opinion from a less experienced surgeon, and does that do us any good at all.* After self-questioning came reality: they would have to leave the state to get an opinion, and by leaving the state they would have to go with a surgeon who was not covered by their insurance provider.

"Ella will have a million-dollar head before this is over," Laurie said out loud to her husband before they got their second opinion, and she wasn't far from the truth. Four or maybe five surgeries add up quickly, and after four or five of them the million-dollar mark really isn't much of a fantasy.

Finally, after reality had set in, after the Darnells decided to face the reality of dealing with insurance if the second opinion seemed like a better option for their daughter than the first opinion of two surgeries, they decided that they would travel to the edges of the earth, even the cold world of Antarctica, and sleep on the stairs of the corporate office of their insurance company to get the surgery covered, and if that didn't happen, to ensure the well-being of their daughter and protect her from more of the slashing mental and emotional effects of surgery, they decided they would rather spend the rest of their lives paying off her million-dollar head than roll the dice again on a fifth surgery—if the second opinion was a better option.

Through research, they found a surgeon in Dr. Fearon in Dallas, who was internationally recognized, extremely well published, and, something that was very important to the Darnells, only worked on heads, and most of his patients were children with craniosynostosis. He had become one of the most recognizable, trusted, and accredited facial surgeon in the country, and maybe the world, in the Darnells' opinion, and few would or could dispute this, and the Darnells knew in their hearts that after meeting with him they would have to stand up, like David in front of the giant Goliath, and fight for the insurance company to pay for the surgery with Dr. Fearon.

Before I walk further into the maze of the insurance journey, it has to be noted that the Darnells insurance company had already approved them for two more surgeries that would cost more than the one surgery, but because the one surgery was not within the provider network, the insurance company was willing to pay more money for two surgeries—more important, the insurance company didn't bat an eye at putting a five-year-old girl beneath the spinning blade of a surgical saw at least two more times and exposing her to all the risks that come with anesthesia, with transfusions, and with rejection of foreign substances in the brain.

When the Darnells left Dr. Fearon's office, their hearts rose in their chests. The heat of the Dallas sun fell down on them outside the Dallas Medical Center in North Dallas. The green, blooming trees from the neighboring park lined the street, and the green grass stretched out westward. He offered them one surgery, and even more refreshing for the parents who had their child's skull bone devoured by an infection of the cement and other foreign substances placed in her skull, he said he could reconstruct her skull using only her bone. They walked out into the North Dallas sun, and on that same trip Ella stood in Cowboys Stadium in Dallas, the home of her parents' favorite NFL team; she wore a big purple Cowboys hat, she ran on the green turf of the field, she lay down on the star in the center of the giant Cowboys helmet at the fifty-yard line, and she held the camera shakily as she took a blurry photo of her mom and dad in the end zone. They knelt down on the helmet in the corner of the end zone. Joe had his arms down at his sides and his Cowboys hat propped above his big smile. Laurie knelt next to him. She wrapped one arm around his back and held his other arm with her hand as she leaned into him. She smiled, even though she was wiped out, tired from Ella's inability to sleep in a hotel room without the comforts of everything she needed to fall asleep. Both Joe and Laurie smiled for that moment, but by the time they walked out of Cowboys Stadium that day they knew that they were embarking on a battle that would not be easily won or possibly would not be won at all.

For nearly the next year, as the surgery date approached, Laurie began a second job: insurance agency warrior. Imagine all the great lawyer movies over the decades—*A Few Good Men, My Cousin Vinny, Philadelphia, Erin Brockovich*—and think about the piles of papers that stacked the protagonist's desk, the long hours and late nights as Tom Hanks or Tom Cruise or Julia Roberts scoured through pages and pages of documents and listen to the frustrating conversations where incompetence, ignorance, and neglect echoed through the theater as you as a moviegoer got frustrated for the protagonist. Now, take away the musical score, with the highs and lows emphasized with sharp changes in tone. And take away the quirky but fun love interest that fuels the protagonist throughout. Oh yeah, and take away the assistants who make great discoveries in the dusty bookshelves in the stacks of the libraries or scan the Internet on the protagonist's behalf. Most important, take away the montages that gloss over months upon months of paper pushing, phone calls, and frustration, because those months, in real-life battles with insurance companies, don't fly by—the winters and springs don't pass and the snows and leaves don't come and go within the span of one perfectly matched song.

Now, add a family. Add a full-time job. Add the special care of a daughter whose head is vulnerable and who can't sleep at night. That was Laurie's life for nearly a year as she fought to get her daughter's surgery covered, fought to cover the surgeon's costs, the anthropologist's cost, the anesthesiologist's cost, the nurse's cost, and all the other costs that would, Laurie hoped, give her daughter the most normal childhood that she could give her, with all the falls and bumps and swings and jumps that accompany childhood. She fought, she fought, and she eventually won.

One week post-op, the Darnells met with the Appeals Board to fight for coverage for Ella's surgery. Ella was a regular energetic three-year-old with a closed skull. A few weeks later, on May 18, 2012, the insurance company approved Ella's surgery with Dr. Fearon. They approved not because a moment of compassion consumed them but because of failed access. But Laurie would take it:

> I'd spent the last 9 months working on this. The battle was time consuming and challenging, but the last few months it has taken a huge toll on me! It's the hardest process I've ever been through! I'm a mama bear and I'm not afraid to ask for and fight for what I feel is best for my little girl! I think I am officially an insurance warrior and I'm proud to say I won my battle! [Laurie said on her blog.] This took a huge toll on all of us. I've been a wreck and I don't handle being lied to! I don't handle lazy people! I don't take NO for an answer very well when it is something I feel passionate about! Ella's health care has been my 2nd job for the last few years and the insurance battle took over as my 3rd job! I'm happy to give up that job and her follow-up appointments will be much fewer! What a relief! Thanks for your support and prayers! I feel like a million pounds was taken off my shoulders today!
>
> I called to tell Joe when I got the great news, and he said, "You did a great job! You worked very hard for this! Can we have the real Laurie back now?"

Like the pro she had become, even though no one would ever want to become such a pro, Ella cruised through pre-op, the meeting with the media representative, the photo shoot, and meetings with the anesthesiologist, the neurosurgeon, and Dr. Fearon. His goal was to do one surgery and only use Ella's bone to close up the gaps in bone in her skull and to do it immediately, two major reasons why Laurie had spent the last nine months of her life calling insurance agencies, harassing incompetent or lazy people who decided to not work on Friday afternoons, and scouring insurance bylaws at the kitchen table with her head between her hands and her elbows on the wooden surface in their kitchen in Salt Lake City.

According to Ella's CT scans, when Dr. Fearon unraveled her skin for the last time he saw the two holes that she was born with like widened eyes on the back of her scalp. He saw ridges of remnants of previous surgeries, with cuts and edges of bone that illustrated Ella's surgical history like a textbook opened to page 1 and thumbed through as his eyes scanned over the cuts and grooves. Then he took all of her bone off again and molded it together. Then she was done. Obviously, the surgery was not that fast, it was not simple, it, like most successful CVRs, was nothing short of a miracle of modern medicine, but it was done, and that was what mattered to the Darnells when they took Ella out of the clinic in North Dallas and brought her back to their hotel room and eventually home to Salt Lake City, where they live at the edge of Rocky Mountains, the cuts and grooves and slants of the giants next to their homes telling the same traumatic history of their growth—just like what lay beneath Ella's skin.

The routine of some melatonin and a Disney movie on the couch to help Ella fall to sleep that was used, initially, to calm the little girl down has become a common practice that has now spanned more than a year's time. Laurie and Joe have tried the same routine in Ella's bed. They set up a TV, tuck her comfortably beneath her blankets, turn the lights down low, sit by her side, and rub her head until she begins to doze off or dozes off completely. Most the time, at the stage when the body begins to let go and the mind begins to relax into sleep Ella fights it and pushes until she finds her way back to the couch, under a blanket, and with Nemo or Woody or a Disney Junior character on the screen. Sometimes, the rarer times, she falls asleep in her bed, the comforts of the blanket, a movie, and her parents' caress too much for her little body to resist. But only minutes after she closes her eyes she wakes scared and runs to the front room or cries until her parents come to get her. With the sound of the TV and Mom and Dad and her little sister within earshot, she can fall asleep. It's the comfort that voices bring, that movement brings, and that the roaming of bodies across the floor brings that nothing else can: the comfort of knowing she is not alone and that her whole family roams around her.

The first surgery, at two years old, began it all. She was handed over to an anesthesiologist and woke up in a recovery room beneath the sterile white blankets and cold metal bars that lined the bed and with nurses and doctors and the beep-beeps of a recovery room. The inability to fall asleep got worse after the second surgery, worse after the third, worse after the fourth, and, yes, worse after the fifth time surgeons did their best to extract, reshape, and replace the skull that pansynostosis had created. The sounds of Ella's family around her let her fall asleep. They give her the comfort that lets her relax her eyes and brain and drift into the night.

Little Ella, at two, three, and four years old, having been through so much surgery in her short life, was scared to fall asleep alone because she was terrified about where she might wake up. She was terrified to close her eyes and wake up in a hospital again.

"My honest feeling is that those many times in the OR changed her. She can't express the why, but it began post-op and continued to get worse after every surgery, so I think she's scared to be alone and scared about what is going to happen after falling asleep," Laurie said as she watched her daughter's body slowly calm down on the couch, the tossing and turning slowing to a mild movement of legs and arms every couple minutes and the sporadic movement of legs and arms slowly stopping until her little girl with the curly brown hair popping out from the top of her blanket begins to breathe heavily and the movement stops and she sleeps.

A year later, Laurie sat down, pulled a pen from her purse, and she thought of all the families who might have to go through what hers had gone through. She thought about their struggles with getting Ella into surgery initially, she thought about the incompetent people or rude people from the insurance company who either brushed her off, forgot about her, or denied her without truly looking at the circumstance, she thought about their sweet doctor who did everything he could for Ella before they decided to go to Dallas to see Dr. Fearon, and she thought about how a year had passed since she won the battle with the insurance companies and since Ella's head had been repaired and it remained solid to that day.

And she wrote to all those families: "You are your child's best advocate. You alone. If you don't look out for what's best for your children, no one will." Then, as the pediatric pharmacist in her took over, she listed all the things parents should do when they first hear that their child has craniosynostosis or any other major problem at birth:

1. Ask questions—there is no stupid question.
    a. Write them down, because you will forget in the appointment.
    b. Write down the answers while in the appointment.
    c. Ask for the best form of communication for further questions (call the office or e-mail).
    d. ALL questions are fair game—this is your CHILD!
2. Remember that a doctor who discourages getting a second opinion is a red-flag.

a. Always ask if this is something that they would recommend a second opinion for.
b. Ask who would be the best person for a local second opinion and ask them who would be the best nationally.
c. Call your insurance company to find other providers covered by your insurance.

3. Do your research.

a. Start with reliable sources on the Internet.
b. Utilize professional Web sites (American Academy of Pediatrics, Mayo Clinic, Medlineplus.gov) and craniosynostosis resources.

4. Remember that you know your child best.

5. Follow your intuition and gut feeling—if something feels wrong, it may be.

6. Phone a friend (or use e-mail or Facebook).

a. Call a friend or family member with a medical background.
b. Reach out to organizations such as CAPPS Kids and Cranio Care Bears.

7. Have a great pediatrician on your side.

a. They can be a valuable resource to help you find the right path of care.
b. They are able to coordinate ALL the care your child is receiving.

8. Don't give up—keep asking questions and bringing your child in if something seems wrong.

9. Write things down and organize a file with the information.

10. Take care of yourself.

Scars

Queen Jocasta recognized her son Oedipus because of the scars on his ankles. His scars defined him, and the thrashings around his ankles symbolized all the hopes of his parents to change what they could not change and to avoid what they could not avoid. Their son would eventually follow the path the oracle set out in front of him, and he would gouge out his eyes in shame. The scars in his eyes would then define him in literature for the millennia to come.

Scarface lived long before Al Pacino lifted his gun in the early eighties and famously said, "Say hello to my little friend." The Blackfoot legend tells the story of Poia, the misplaced son of Morning Star and the grandson of the sun and moon. Poia was half human and half god and because of his mother's, Feather Woman's, foolishness he had been banned from the heavens. Poia (meaning "Scarface") hid from strangers and ran from footsteps, and he had a big scar scratched across his face. People ridiculed him and persecuted him for his ugliness, so he sought out his grandparents, the sun and the moon, and they took pity on him, removed his scar, and taught him the sun dance. He returned to his people with a face clean of scars and taught them the sun dance. They forever adored him. His scar defined him and the removal of it redefined him.

At one time, scars were seen as trophies. Ares, the god of war, ran to Zeus to show off the scars he gained in battle. Morning Star, Poia's father, could be seen as the Blackfoot god of war and the ruler of the thunderbolt and happy to have been scarred, and Indra, the Hindu god of the thunderbolt, bore a deep scar across his face. Those with scars wielded power and honor. They rode through the heavens and their scars shone as symbols of the bravery, all manifestations of the Zimbabwe saying "A coward has no scars."

In Western civilization, however, those with scars are seen as villains. The Joker's scars rip from the edges of his lips—people turn from his hideousness.

In the newest film in the Batman series, *The Dark Knight*, the Joker, beautifully done by the late Heath Ledger, plays with people's curiosity by asking, "I bet you'd like to know how I got these scars?" He changes his answer every time he answers the question—each time he reveals a more sinister and evil story. The scars that tear up his face and are covered by bright red makeup define him, as do the scars of other great villains whom we in Western culture love to hate—Scar from *The Lion King*, Freddy Krueger, the previously mentioned Pacino character, Frankenstein's monster, Craterface from *Grease*, Two-Face— the list goes on and on. But this phenomenon of defining evil with red and raised skin is not new. *The Guardian* recently published an article listing the most famous scarred literary villains that showed, at least within Western culture, that authors have been pinning the scar on the villain for centuries.

Although it is debatable, there is a full school of thought that believes that we, as humans, do not like scars because a facial scar disrupts the symmetrical aesthetic for which we biologically yearn. Many point to Plato's golden proportions as the seminal thought that led to the studies of symmetry and beauty. A scar has no place on a symmetrical face. It throws off our natural love of a balance. This theory of symmetry and its tie to beauty extends past the face and has been found to be plausibly true in symmetry of bodies: the more symmetrical the body, the more desirable. So those with scars are not only battling a social stigma but a biological stigma as well.

We're all scarred one way or another. I bear the scar of a forgotten surgery on a forgotten day from a forgotten doctor. It runs the length of my head and makes me fear things that come too close to my face. I've covered it up for nearly twenty years, and now it peeks out from beneath my stringy and thinning hair.

Last night I had a dream, the same dream that makes me smile while I sleep but makes me sad when I wake. In the dream, hair covers my scalp and there are no recessions that run from the worry lines on my forehead to the back of my head. It's silly, but it's always the same—I style my hair in different ways: faux hawks and spiky and business casual with it all parted to one side. Then I stare into the mirror and ask my reflection why he worried so much and for so many years. Then I wake up and place a finger on my scar, not having to push hair out of the way to get to touch it, and I fall back asleep with the hope that I can dream (live) a few more hours with a full head of hair and forget about my scar. Then I realize that these worries of mine are so superficial. These problems I've created for myself are nothing compared to those of people with much more serious diseases and who are stricken with scars that don't just remind them of past pathologies like mine but predict their futures. Those with cancer, with heart disease, those who suffered strokes, those with scars that tell how they will eventually die or had almost died. I have to say right here, right now, that I will never compare myself to those who have dealt or will deal with much worse than I ever had to deal with—only the mothers will know.

The Shave

Twelve years later, I finally took her up on her offer to love me with scars and all. Mary, my wife of nine years and mother of our beautiful two-year-old boy, held a mirror in front of my face, and I held shears in my hand and looked up at the mirror, ready to drag the rotating blades across the little hair that I had left and shave my head for the first time in my life. We set up the shearing station outside our house on a way-too-hot day in early September 2013. While my hairline had receded drastically and the only hair left on my forehead in front of my scar popped out of the evenly spaced hair plugs, dark and thick hair that stood out against my skin, it was enough to cover what it was originally put there to cover. Mary held the mirror in front of me. I held the shears at the edge of my fake hairline and began.

A flash of sunlight reflected off the mirror and made me blink. If it weren't for that brief flash of too-bright light, I don't know if I would have given the act of shaving one last thought, but I did, briefly, wondering if I really needed to shave my head to complete the abstract journey of finding the real me beneath the hair. I'd begun to sweat in the heat, and the sweat fell down around my ears. Mary held the mirror in front of me, and she nodded at me and gave me a half smile. With that, I plunged the clippers into the center of my thinning front hairline.

I'd thought about my hairline every day of my life since I started to lose it in the mid–1990s and thought about it even more since the day the plastic surgeon took a line of hair from the back of my head and put it up front. *What if people know? What if they think I was just worried about going bald? What if they think I'm shallow? Does it really look that bad?* My thoughts drifted more toward the plugs than they did toward the scars, and as I dragged the clippers across my head, my hair fell down onto my shoulders. I buzzed an inch backward on my forehead until I found the start of my scar. I followed it and

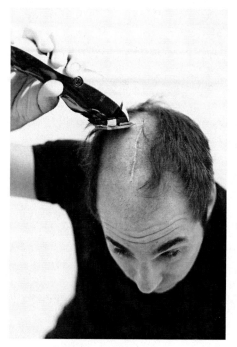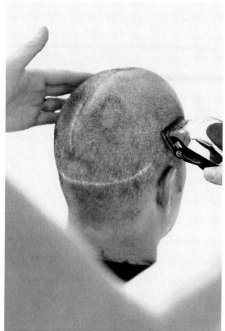

My first shave in my lifetime (courtesy of Heather Bird Photography).

expected it to follow a straight line to the back of my head and end at the back, the top of my skull. It did not. It weaved back and forth in little jagged turns from the front to the back to the left and weaved its way through what I saw to be more visually telling than the scar: bumps and bends and slants that rose and fell and dipped. From straight ahead, my head looked like it came to a point on the left side like a tilted cone that had fallen to one side. In short: it's one big slant.

The bright white skin of a scalp that had never seen the sun shone bright and pale against my dark hair like a river of dry white sand flowing between shady trees. The pattern of plugs sat evenly spaced and triangular on the top of my forehead, and from the top it looked like the triangular shape of my forehead when I was born, the plugs unnaturally forming a point, just like my closed sagittal suture, on the top of my head.

The long, wavy scar fell farther back than I had thought it would. It kept going until it nearly touched the scar created for the transplant. When I had finally shaved all the hair off, with two mirrors, one in front of me and one behind me, I saw the back of my head clean and shaved for the first time. The second scar sharply cut into my skin from ear to ear and formed a slight downward bow. The two together formed a white anchor in an already-white ocean of skin, and I felt free of everything for a brief moment, free of the worries of people thinking about why I tried so hard to cover my head, free of all the people who said, "Why don't you just shave it? You'll look better," free of wondering about how people thought of me, and free of my worries about my hair, natural and replaced, like the anchor that fell across the back of my head.

I ran my hands over my fuzzy head and felt the mix of hot sunlight and cool sweat on my scalp, a sensation I had never had before. I massaged both scars and it felt good. Then I found the bathroom mirror and saw the lumps and bumps that made up my shaven head. I was shocked at how visually mellow the scar was and how shocking the bumps and slants and curves were. The little hair I had, had done a good job with those bumps and slants and curves, and for a moment I wished for it back. After I took the straight razor to the tiny hairs that were left after the clippers had done their job, my head looked like a cantaloupe from the back with the veins of the fruit running the white, white rind of the not so perfectly round melon.

Mary sat me down on the toilet seat and finished the job with the straight razor. She tugged and pulled at the last bits of remaining hair until I was clean all the way around. Then she wiped the shaving cream off my head with a towel and smiled at me.

"I'm glad it's finally done," she said. There were scores of reasons why she said it. The main one, I guessed, was because I had talked about it off and on for years, more frequently the last few months, and nonstop for the week after I had decided exactly when I would shave it off.

"What do you think?" I asked her. I've never been told I have a puppy dog look, but in my mind's eye that's what I was giving her.

"It looks good," she said. She knew and I knew that she was in a very tough spot. She knew that no matter what she said, my insecurity, worrying mind, and critical approach to tone and inflection would hammer at it until she stopped talking because I would take everything negatively.

"What do you mean, 'good'?" I asked her immediately.

She closed her eyes and smiled a bit, searching for patience with a paranoid husband.

"It looks fine, Kase," she said. "I mean, for everything they did to your head, it looks good. The lumps are bigger than I thought they would be and the scar is actually lighter, but it's your head, ya know." She gave me a hug, hoping that I had really listened to her and didn't break down every syllable, every shift in pitch, and every word. And I did my best not to.

I hugged her back and stood up to take one last long look at it before the whole scene would end. I didn't really recognize myself in the mirror. And, to be honest, I wished I could have loved what I saw when I stood there and looked in the mirror. I wanted to love my head as it was. I wanted to embrace it immediately and forget all the years of worry, the mornings covering up my scalp with my thinning hair and the old lady in church nearly twenty years earlier who told me to take my hat off. But, at first, right there in our bathroom, the lumps and slants and sharp valleys that fell down to my scar were too much for me, too much for someone like me, with a vanity and fear of what others might think.

"Your hat's on the kitchen table. Now, let's go get lunch."

She threw her purse around her shoulder and headed out the front door, forcing me away from the mirror and away from the morning.

After lunch I decided to text my mom and dad and warn them. Most of the time, growing up and in our adulthood, my brother and I did whatever we could to shock our mom with snakes, with crude jokes, or with anything else that might make her gasp, but with this news I wanted to ease her into it, spare her feelings as much as I could. I know one person thought about craniosynostosis, even though she never knew the medical term before I learned it and shared it with her in 2010, more than I did, and it was my mom.

"I shaved my head this morning," I texted my mom and dad. There was no need to fill them in on why it was so important.

They both texted back immediately but separately, my dad from work and my mom from home.

MOM: "What? Why did you decide to do that?"

DAD: "How'd it go?"

ME: "I did it for photos for the book." I thought this might be easier than texting them about confronting my demons, accepting myself for who I am, and shedding twenty years of worry off my back—it would be tough to punctuate all of that, and they didn't need to hear about it either. They had always made decisions to protect me and to make my life easier. Even now as I write this, I know they will read it, and I want to save their feelings.

MOM: "How are the scars? Pictures!"

ME: "They're not bad. It's pretty lumpy up there though." I attached a photo, one from the front of my head where all they could see was my smile and a slight unevenness of my skull.

DAD: "I think you look wiser and more professional."

MOM "How's the back scar?"

ME: "Worse than the original."

MOM: "Yeah, that wasn't a good idea." Right there. We were on the same page—relief.

ME: "Love you guys!"

For the first time since the transplant, they had admitted that we all made the wrong decision and this, more than nearly anything else that day for some odd reason, made me feel better, like we had joined some sort of team together in our regret at covering up something that had not only shaped my exterior but also shaped my personality, giving me a strong stroke of insecurity that runs so deeply through me I could never dig it out, and my relationship with my mom and dad, as they still look at me as their baby who was so sick as a newborn as he lay in the incubator for months and waited for his body to hold on to ten pounds so the doctors could take him away, open up his skull, place him in some kind of something that would dissolve over time, and then bandage him up before placing him back in their arms.

DAD: "We love your head."

MOM: "See you tomorrow. Love you."

I would see my mom a few days later. She would glance briefly at my head before I put my hat back on and shove the whole experience somewhere deep inside of her without letting it sink in. My dad, much taller than me, would wrap his arms around my bald head and give my head a hug. We talked very little about it after that. Maybe it was because I didn't want to make more of a big deal about it than I already had. Maybe it was because they didn't either. Maybe it was because we'd talked about my damn head so much over the last year and a half since I started interviewing people and maybe because each time I had shared from those interviews my mom had teared up with empathy for the families who had to go through what she went through. Or maybe it was because there was nothing more to say, like the cycle had finally been completed. The only thing my mom would say to me after I shaved my head was, "Wow, it grows back fast." And I'm okay with whatever she's okay with.

Later in the day, after Mary and I had spent the day together and she had to assure me fifty times that I looked all right, due to my silliness that I regret now, I thought about all those who have no choice in keeping their hair, because of cancer—two days after I shaved my head one of my good friends, after months of chemotherapy, had a double mastectomy to remove a tumor that had ravaged her at the old age of thirty-seven years—which gave me the necessary perspective. I will always be the child who had the surgery and doesn't remember the pain. We, the children with craniosynostosis, for the most part, just have to deal with how the birth defect shaped us physically and without a doubt mentally, but again, for the most part, we don't have to deal with worry, the memories, the thought of losing a child—that has been reserved for our parents and, it seems, especially reserved for the hearts and minds of our mothers.

Even so, when Mary and I picked up our son from day care that day, I had my hat snug tight on my head. The cool texture of the cloth on my bare head and the sweat beads that dripped down to the edge of the hat reminded me without the need to think about it that I would look different to him. Since the day he was born, he has been a thinker, a concentrator, and an observer. He'd always been so serious when something new came his way. As a baby, he would sit and hold his toys and wrap his fingers around them and touch them with each end of his fingertips until he had scanned every crevice of brightly colored plastic. As a one-year-old boy he would get frustrated if every item on his high chair wasn't perfectly placed in its allotted slot, and as a toddler, with the eye of a surveyor, he scans and thinks and stares at a new environment before moving forward into it with caution. There was no way he wasn't going to notice the scars and bumps that had come to the surface of his father's head that morning. I worried about this for some reason.

"Will he recognize me without hair?" I asked Mary on the way to day care. "Will the scars be weird to him?"

"You still have your same old face," she said. Then she giggled at my insecurities.

We picked him up and headed home where the games always began.

I sat on the couch, watched him play, and made noises with my mouth until he came running to me at full two-year-old speed, legs fumbling for a couple steps and then catching a bit of rhythm and then fumbling over each other again until he lunged onto my lap and I picked him up to kiss his cheek. It took less than a second to say "hat" and grab the bill of the brown hat I had stolen from my college-bound nephew and pull it off my head. Unlike before, it stuck and pulled as my sticky head tried to hold on to it.

Lukas threw my hat on the ground, and in his surveying way he found my scars and bumps immediately. He ran his little fingers along my scalp and looked at them as they touched my skin. I just watched his eyes. They moved up and down and from side to side until he looked down at mine and said with a giggle, "Daddee," as if I had done this for his amusement, like when I say good-bye and walk into the wall and fall down for him. Then he smiled, giggled again, and hugged my head.

Release

Tara Pendleton, in a quiet room in the PICU of the NYU Medical Center, turns on the microphone. Her voice is shaken. It trembles, but she persists. The only sound that can be heard as she begins to speak is the guttural rasp of her voice.

"I'm sitting in the hospital with Cameron. He has come out from surgery and is in the PICU. It has been a very long day. The surgery was delayed by several hours. Leading up to that point was very difficult. My emotions were all over the place. Today was strange with my emotions. My level of sadness of fear for the surgery itself as it was for Cameron, just knowing what he was going to be going through, just sad, in general, that he has to go through that," she says.

For the most part she and her husband were calm before the surgery. They had prayed through the night and come up with the same answer that Tara had believed from the beginning: that Cameron needed to be operated on. Her heart knew this.

She sits in the silent PICU room and whispers into the microphone like it has become her friend, her confidant that she uses to spare her husband and family and friends from the millions of worries that cloud and suffocate her thoughts—they hear enough already, she believes. At the end of each sentence, her voice rises like the swell of a wave finally cresting and landing onshore. The first parts of her sentences roll like swelling sadness, but by the time her last word comes out there is a hope that rings so clearly from her mouth. Her happiness comes from one thing. For months and months and years upon years, from ICP test to ICP test in Ohio, the doctors told her and her husband Shawn, that Cameron had no indication of ICP, that there was no pressure sitting on his brain, that all was fine, and that his brain had enough room to grow without the pressing of the skull against it. Her hope and happiness lived in that as her five-year-old son lay next to her in the PICU bed, a young boy, not an infant like most who undergo the surgery. His ophthalmologist report and other reports showed no ICP.

"I have a lot of feelings about these reports. The tests are simply not accurate," Tara says. "Surgeons cannot use this as a guide. I'm so thankful that he lays next to me and is on the other side." Her voice moves slowly in small changes of tone and pitch from happiness with sadness to happiness with anger when she talks about her previous surgeon consultations and their reliance on the ICP tests. Then her voice shifts to triumph.

At 5:30 in the recording, Cameron wakes. He whimpers for a moment like a wounded cub. The whimper is soft at first but then turns to a cry, a cry that shoots through the silent room and breaks Tara's thought mid-sentence. There is silence again. Complete silence without her voice. Cameron spent most of his time in the PICU in extreme discomfort. The medications for pain didn't work well for him, didn't calm him down, and his cries and moans and whimpers crawled out from beneath his swollen eyes and bandages.

"My eyes hurt," he tells his parents. His father, not a surgeon or other medical professional, did what he knew to do. He asked the nurses for ice packs, he placed them gently on his son's eyes, and the crying and whimpering stopped until the packs had to be swapped out, and during those few moments while his father takes off the old packs and replaces them Cameron cries and whimpers again, lying uncomfortably and, at age five, old enough to know that the pain is pain.

"I'm sorry, but my son is crying," she says into the microphone. "But I have to tell mothers this while I am here in this moment." She goes silent again, a rustling sound is heard, and Cameron's tears stop just long enough for her to say, "I'm telling you this now because I want all mothers to know that their motherly instinct is the most powerful tool they have and to listen to it." The recorder clicks off after a small whimper from her boy and the sound of what can only be described as lips touching skin.

Mornings. I am, of course, stopped by sounds or words. They may come from a mother or a father or from the cry of a child, but some words hold on stronger than others, make me stop typing, push me away from my computer and into the real world to breathe in life without craniosynostosis at its center. Delving multiple times into the lives of families who have struggled and been torn apart and sewn back together by craniosynostosis, repeated surgeries, skeptical surgeons, and unwanted surgical outcomes is emotionally difficult, but I have gotten better at compartmentalizing emotion and writing—as long as I keep the image of my mom at twenty-seven years old and the tears from the mothers I've met out of mind.

Most mornings, I wake up, roll out of bed, make my standard fare of toast with peanut butter, fill my cup with coffee, and head downstairs to read someone else's words before crossing my fingers and beginning to hammer out some of my own prose. With some luck, I will resurface before the sun comes up and start my day, either teaching or grading or watching my son. Sometimes my luck is good, and sometimes it is not. This is the life of a writer. And I am tired after writing.

This morning, in particular, I sit and listen to a recording of one of the families for the book. In the quiet of my basement office, only the company of overgrown branches looking into my window, with my tiny, round and gray space heater kicking out a warming breath, I listen. For all but two families for the book, I met them face-to-face. I walked into their homes, shook their hands, tried to shake off my nerves, set up my recorder and listened. But this morning, I listen to a recording from one of the two families I didn't get to meet, so I have no idea what will be coming next.

There are tears. There are coughs to hopefully cover the tears. But I imagine the family sitting around the recorder like they are trying to imagine me in it, a little grown man with craniosynostosis on the other side. They've done a very good job narrating their story, as they are in the thick of decision making and waiting for their child to go into surgery, but as if tears and fear make a sound, their voices crack and the shuffle of the clothes, I imagine, is them wiping away their tears.

Then. A mother is alone. She has turned the recorder on. A draft pushes through the door of my basement office, the only barrier between me and the three-degree weather of early December in Utah.

"I don't want to burden my family any more than they are already burdened with my worries," she says in a whisper. This whisper came out of my speakers like a shout. She sniffles, pulling the excess mucus that accompanies tears back. "So I will tell you, my little friend."

Those words stopped me—"my little friend." Something in them pushed me backward in retreat like a scared dog who had been beaten too many times by an owner when his owner raises his hand to pet him. For a moment, my body was swarmed by anxiety, warming at the temples and swirling in the belly. And I became afraid of the responsibility I had been given by this woman and, now I understand, by all the mothers and fathers who let me into their lives to tell their stories and for some, like her, to be a confidant.

I have been told by many that it is so nice to see me all grown-up after having my surgery nearly forty years ago. I've had mothers, my age and younger, run their hands over my head and hug me as if I were their child thirty-seven years in the future. Because I teach at a university, some have showered me with love because I have become a successful part of society, and since I do teach at the college level they believe that I am intelligent—I try to act the part when I am with them, more to create a sense of confidence in a man who will write about their journey than to seem smarter than I really am.

"So I will tell you, my little friend," however, hit me with more of an awakening to my important part in all of this than I had ever thought I had.

I push myself away from my chair and walk upstairs with the excuse to get coffee, not to run away from those words spoken into a microphone. Frost covers the window over the kitchen sink. Wings of cold created art on the glass, flowing down and then back up like giant frozen snowflakes on what used to be hot sand. *Frosty the Snowman* plays on the TV in the living room, and my two-year-old son hears me rattling around in the kitchen with the coffeepot. He stomps around the corner, barely missing his head on the corner of the countertop, and looks up at me and says, "Happy birthday." He is not really saying "happy birthday" to me but actually quoting Frosty's first words from the 1960s TV special. Lukas doesn't even smile but just plods back out of the room.

"Good morning, buddy," I say. I wish I could sit with him on my lap and watch that animated show for the one hundredth time this holiday season and not worry about what I need to do in the basement, but I fill my coffee cup and walk back down the stairs, through the could basement, and into my semi-heated office.

I rewind the recording. "My little friend."

What do these families see in me? Who am I to them? I ask myself before I start to write again. The last few months have been hard to write. But this morning these words that stop me have gotten me started again, but this time with an even deeper understanding of why.

* * *

Just a few days before Cameron's surgery, Tara stood next to her line of suitcases and packed for the trip to New York City. She folded clothes and tucked them into the corners of bags. Shawn's collared shirts. Her pants. Socks. Extra shoes. All the stuff needed for the three of them to make it through more than a week on the road, in a hotel room, and in the PICU before coming back home. Her emotions got the best of her that day. Her worry about his future and her and her husband's decision. Part of her said that she would keep Cameron how he is because she loved every ounce of her five-year-old boy, but the other side of her told her how selfish that would be and that she would be hurting his chance at a normal life.

Her tears, as she stood alone in her room and packed, fell down onto Cameron's shirts when she packed them too into the corners of the suitcase. Some of them were normal, full of the colors and designs that five-year-olds like to wear. But some of them were not so normal—they still had all the markings of a young boy, but Tara had surgery performed on them. She enlisted the help of a friend to sew invisible zippers on them for Cameron's head to slide through after surgery. After the cutting was done, she sewed in zippers on the edges of the cuts from the collar of the shirt so that she could unzip the shirt after surgery and slide the large, extended remade collar over his head without hurting him or touching the bandages. Her idea for the zipper, although this was the first time she had actually made a zipper shirt for him, didn't grow in the moments of fear once the surgery had been scheduled. It grew many months—and maybe years—earlier when Cameron first started to complain that it hurt when she pulled his T-shirts over his elongated head. T-shirts' collars just aren't made for boys with the boat-like-shaped head created by sagittal craniosynostosis, although she could never get a doctor to agree that the boy's head needed to be surgically repaired, not his T-shirts.

* * *

The Pendletons took a much longer path to surgery than most families, and instead of "took" it would be better described as "blazed" a different path with the hatchets of determination, fear, and self-doubt. In the last week of July, Cameron, a three-year-old boy who was very good at being a three-year-old boy, tipped a motorized toy Jeep and fell on his head. His eyes broadened, he was sick to his stomach, and his mental awareness dropped, all symptoms of a concussed brain. The ER doctors wanted to make sure he didn't do anything more to his brain with the fall, so they took some CT scans and found the fall hadn't done any real damage, maybe because his head had a thick layer of bone where his sagittal suture should have been—it had closed way too early, as the sagittal suture usually remains open for many years. When Tara heard this, she knew that there had always been something "off" about her third son's head, because she had two older boys to compare it with.

There had been three years of well visit appointments with their pediatrician, who, when Tara pointed to the boat-like shape of Cameron's head, just laughed it off as a mother worrying too much because mothers worry too much.

"I think it looks like an alien shape or maybe, or maybe a football or ET," Tara told her pediatrician. This all came from a kind woman and a loving mom who wanted the pediatrician to take her concerns seriously—because objectifying Cameron's head tore through her like a swallowed blade.

"He's fine. He'll grow into it." The pediatrician laughed.

From the ER, after Cameron's tipping of the Jeep, the Pendletons were sent to see the plastic surgeon. Fear. Confirmation of past worries. The plastic surgeon wanted to perform the surgery, but he urged them to take the wait-and-see approach to Cameron's head, and Shawn agreed. He didn't see Cameron's head to be as misshapen as Tara did. Shawn didn't think Cameron's head looked all that bad and agreed that a visit to the neurosurgeon should determine the need for surgery, because both parents, at the time, agreed that they would not do this for "cosmetic" reasons. Both parents felt this would be the right path when they left the plastic surgeon's office. They were told that Cameron had a mild case and that his head would look about the same as he aged but just a larger version of the same head, one that, both parents would agree, wasn't that bad.

"I mean I have a pretty large forehead." Shawn laughed. "He could have just been my son."

"If everything neurologically was okay, we would not go through surgery," Tara said.

Shawn, a very even man, even though his first instinct was to opt out of surgery because the "cosmetic" diagnosis was not enough, started to think about all of those visits to the pediatrician as well. He thought of his older boys and how Cameron seemed to have dropped behind them in development, how their pediatrician, when asked about Cameron's speech delays, looked at him with eyes that said, *He's three* or *He's four. What do you want me to do?* Those things, happening in the background, started to surface in Shawn's mind and meld with those that had risen long ago in Tara's, but the two were agreed: no surgery just to make him look better, despite the fact that both Shawn and Tara knew Cameron was falling behind developmentally.

Our minds are powerful when we want to believe something, especially when that something seems the better option of two. When a pain shoots through our gut, we want to blame the spicy foods and ignore the other symptoms of something worse. When we drink too much and the morning after slams down on our foreheads with pains from dehydration and deprival, we want to blame the light dinner we had before drinking glass after glass of red wine. Denial is a beast that can devour our logical thoughts. It climbs over our weak walls of mental fortitude that were put up to keep the truth safe from the attack of emotions and hope. Denial too, however, comes from ignorance, not the kind of ignorance that stems from lack of education or knowledge but the kind of ignorance that grows out of the fear of not knowing what to do with that education or knowledge—like the pediatrician not sending the

Pendletons to the neurosurgeon because he didn't know what to do with the slight misshapenness of Cameron's head—and it roots itself deeply and sprouts strong limbs that fight off even the strongest of gut feelings or intuition that point to the worse of the two options. Sometimes.

"We were told at that time that it was a risky surgery for an older child," said Tara.

"We were told continually that there were no reasons for his delays. All the specialists told us over and over that they saw no signs of problems from the sagittal synostosis. No extra fluid in the brain. No intercranial pressure," Sean said. A slight guffaw fell from his mouth, the kind of release of air that comes from frustration, as he and his wife sat and waited for their son's surgery in the upcoming month, and unlike the other parents in this book, there is no softening through time with the Pendletons. Their story, their words, their worries, come full force, two parents in the thick of their spinning thoughts about the spinning blades of major cranial reconstructive surgery for a boy who will probably remember it all. There's more blood loss with older kids. The brain is much less malleable. The complications are much higher at an older age and Cameron was way beyond the point of easy modification of cranial bones.

"Hold on, wait, let's see if symptoms come. See you in six months." These words sickened Tara's stomach, tore through her motherly instincts, ate at her intuition. Then, more than a year later in the summer of 2012, Cameron, four years old, woke multiple times in the middle of the night, walked into his parents' room, climbed into their bed, snuggled up to his mom and dad, pointed to one spot on the front of his head, and asked, "Mommy, why does my head always hurt right here?"

"Most likely allergies," would be the neurosurgeon's typical response.

Then the change came on, not organically but with immediacy. A happy toddler became aggressive. He stopped meeting milestones. It turned on a dime. It wasn't temper tantrums. The Pendletons with two older boys knew what those were. But Cameron became meaner.

In June of 2012 they sought a second opinion from a plastic surgeon and a neurosurgeon. Tara was nervous. But she was certain something had to be done. She was scared of surgery, but she was dealing with the daily fear of the symptoms that might come on: blindness (loss of vision), migraines, and developmental disabilities.

The second opinion was different but no better.

"Cameron's very mild," the neurosurgeons said.

"No intercranial pressure," said the ophthalmologist.

Tara coughs and talks. "As the mother, I had a different feeling." It wasn't until the Pendletons consulted another plastic surgeon that someone finally told them that the ICP tests, he believed, were inconclusive tests, as some children who tested low had high pressure when opened up and some who showed high pressure on the tests when opened up had very low pressure. Shawn, however, as many would feel, played the conservative role. He believed that when it came to major cranial surgery the doctors knew what they were talking about.

"So when are you going to be okay with a doctor's answer?" Shawn asked Tara repeatedly. In his mind, he wondered if Tara would only be satisfied when surgery was the answer. He asked her if there would ever be a right answer from doctors, and Tara, admittedly, asked herself the same questions. Did she believe something was wrong with Cameron because she watched through a magnifying glass every day, watching every misstep, hearing every verbal inconsistency or oddity, and tying them to his sagittal synostosis? And she asked herself if it was just her rise in anxiety that brought on the incessant research into the birth defect and the hours on the Internet looking at children with craniosynostosis that only led her to babies who were operated on—and this find only made the worries worse for her. She couldn't find any children Cameron's age. She couldn't find out if their symptoms came on like his. She couldn't find out if they had complications. She couldn't find anything. The anxiety grew. Then Tara found help. She found Amy Galm at CAPPS Kids. And Amy led the Pendletons to the team of Dr. Staffenberg and Dr. Weiner in New York City. The Pendletons flew to New York City.

Tara woke the next morning in an apartment across from NYU Medical. She woke with what she believed was the answer to her husband's question. She was anxious, but it was a good anxious, and she believed that whatever Dr. Staffenberg diagnosed she would be at peace with.

"The journey thus far has not been a good one, and I'm looking forward to a new journey. I'm very confident that Dr. Staffenberg will help my son. And I cannot live my life and not help my son. I can't sit by and wait for symptoms that will change my son's life for the worse. And not to mention the cosmetic part. I don't want my son teased. I don't want my son bullied. I want him to have the best quality of life possible for him," Tara, her voice nervous and jittery, said as she looked across at NYU from their apartment by the East River, where I had sat to wait and talk to the same man only months earlier.

"I didn't wish the symptoms on my boy, but I wish they would have come earlier. I would never wish to make him go through any of that, but we might have been able to have surgery earlier. It would have made everything easier. I know that sounds awful to say," Shawn said.

Shawn, beginning in April after their consultation with Dr. Staffenberg and Dr. Weiner, made his way alongside Tara, and they both stared at the future together and asked the hard questions that come with the other option. What if Cameron had debilitating headaches his whole life? What happened if he lost vision at sixteen years old? What happened if he was so disfigured that he pulled away from life? What if the symptoms got worse? What if the world treated him differently even if he was normal? Was it just cosmetic? Was it their vanity?

Their worries about the term "cosmetic" were not new to the craniosynostosis world. Most parents who have an option to operate have to suffer through all the feelings and doubts that the word "cosmetic" evokes. However, as the Pendletons' surgeon Dr. Staffenberg believes, the word "cosmetic" should no longer be associated with the fixing of craniosynostosis:

> Chances are if there's no tested increase in ICP, some doctors will say, "This is really just a cosmetic problem." If I were a young parent, and a doctor told me this, I would feel terrible for even considering putting my baby through an operation that sounds like it's really my vanity ... and so "cosmetic," as a plastic surgeon, I see as a really bad word to use, and you know, there's no question that this reconstruction we're talking about is because the forehead or head shape is not anywhere in the realm of normal. It attracts attention. There's no question about it, and so what we're doing is we're reconstructing the skull or the forehead so that we're taking something that is not in the range of normal and putting it in the range of normal. Where "cosmetic" would be taking something normal and somehow trying to improve upon it.
>
> The idea that young parents are being told that a triangular-shaped forehead is really a cosmetic problem is unfair to them because it's now making them feel guilty, so I think that the right way to look at this for us is that there's no question that this is a reconstructive problem, not a cosmetic problem, but the results or the quality of the reconstruction is partially being judged by that cosmetic merit [Dr. Staffenberg explained].
>
> "We don't want our baby to go through school with a stigma." "We don't want people making assumptions about what the baby can or can't do." "We don't want, you know, our son, when he's old enough to play football, to have to get a custom-made helmet to fit." You know, we have patients like this that can't fit into a bike helmet, that can't do what normal people do, and why wasn't surgery done? Because ... [parents] were told it was just a cosmetic problem. You know, it's a bad word to use because we all make the same sort of subconscious ... we draw the same conclusions. Can you imagine how many babies would be judged differently because of their head shape? They could have normal intelligence. But because of your abnormality, you would be seen as slow? [he asks the question]. That's just unfair [Dr. Staffenberg reiterates].

A man, whose name I cannot tell, told me stories that I didn't want to hear, and if it were up to me, even if he were okay with me sharing his name,

I wouldn't want to because I fear that someone who reads this will see him as an isolated case when his stories are emblematic of many, many people like him and if he were seen as an isolated case, which may happen if I name him, families may not listen to his story and advice, thinking, *That could not happen to my child.* There is a certain kind of truth that comes from knowing no one can point to you as the storyteller, and there is a certain kind of honesty that comes from a man who is brave enough to tell his story but isn't looking for notoriety, and this man has given me truths and honesty without asking for anything in return. So emblematic is his story of people who were born just years before me, who were never diagnosed with craniosynotosis, sagittal synostosis in his case, that where I have changed the details of his life to conceal his identity I have only substituted details of place and time—not narratives—that would be true of another person's life, who was undiagnosed, from that place and time. And there will be no description of him in these pages, as he was uncomfortable sharing photos, which, if I understand few things on this journey, this I understand.

Born in the early 1970s, just a few years after surgery for the release of sutures had become very common and just a few years before I was born, this man was born with sagittal synostosis and went undiagnosed as an infant and didn't realize or know what he was born with, just knowing that he was born with something wrong with his skull. Watching a Discovery Channel show, one nearly two decades old, he saw the reconstruction of people's skulls who had major deformities and finally learned what was the cause of his elongated head, but he wasn't actually diagnosed until his son was born.

In the moments before they released this man's wife and his newborn son from the hospital after his birth, this man asked the doctors if they were going to refer his son to a specialist for his elongated head, his craniosynostosis.

"Oh, that's just from the birth canal," the doctors told him. "That will go away."

The man removed his cap to reveal his elongated—boat-shaped—head and said, "I've been waiting thirty years for this to go away." He diagnosed his son, having done his research after watching the Discovery Channel program. The nurse just looked at him, dumbfounded, and released the family that day without ever taking his diagnosis seriously. From there, the man and his wife told their pediatrician what was happening to their son. They had to do all the legwork, and they had to make their own appointments with specialists to get their son's corrective surgery. But no matter what, their son would have surgery.

"As someone who lives with this, there is nothing cosmetic about this surgery," he said. "In school, as a boy, since my head was different they put me in remedial classes." Teachers would walk up to him as a child, they would look at his head, they would remove him from the general population of students, and they would insist that since his head was shaped so oddly he had to have learning or developmental or mental disabilities, so he spent his school years being excluded from other students because of the way he looked, not because of his test scores, so when he reads about doctors using the word "cosmetic" to describe the surgery he laughs a guttural laugh filled with anger at the word's usage, because "as someone who lives with this, there is nothing cosmetic about this surgery."

As a little boy, without the knowledge we have as adults, he followed the teachers into those remedial groups and he, for the most part, remained unaware of his segregation until it ran up to him and slapped him in the face in front of all of his classmates, and from that point it never left him, a revelation that could not be unrevealed.

One day during the middle of a second- or third-grade classroom, his teacher brought in and set up a video camera. This was new. Cameras had finally been whittled down to a size that teachers could carry in their hands and set up on a tripod in the corner of the room, like this boy's teacher did that day. Students sat around tables and talked about the subject of the day, which happened to be bullying in school. While the room rumbled with chatter, each student got the chance to get behind the video camera and turn it, move it to focus on different parts of the room and the conversations. When it came to be this boy's turn, he walked behind the camera and filmed the students and teachers as they talked about bullying.

One young, kind girl spoke as if the boy had left the room. "I don't know how he does it," she said. "I mean, even the teachers attack him, but he just keeps going. I don't think I could."

The boy, standing behind the camera and watching and listening to what she said, felt that self-awareness that he stood outside of everyone else, outside of the group that talked at the table, not only because he stood behind the protection of the camera but also because his head was different.

"When you make a mistake as a person with a disability," he said to me, and then clarified that he meant a "perceived disability," as his intelligence level is very high, "you have to start all over. When a normal person makes a mistake, it's just a mistake. When I made mistakes, I had to prove to everyone again that I wasn't retarded." His voice trails off for a moment. "But like that girl said, I've been known for just keeping going. I don't quit."

There is nothing cosmetic about this, he said, before telling me about a time that serves as a microcosm of his life of being picked on from a young age and being called and treated like a "retard" every day of his life.

Just after the turn of millennium he, working as a heavy equipment engineer on a construction job site, looked across the road. His gaze fell upon another building site where some of the newest, most beautiful and envied heavy equipment stood on the ground out front of the foreman's office. He walked across the street and into the foreman's office and asked if he would consider him as a new heavy equipment engineer. He told the foreman about his more than twelve years' experience, his exemplary record, and his flat-out desire to work with the new equipment that towered outside the door.

"Well, I only hire union," the foreman said.

It didn't take long for the man to go to the union office, sign up, and pay his dues. When the union handed him his first ticket, as luck would have it, he got a ticket to work on the site where he had been told to become a union member to be considered.

He walked in, excited to begin working for his new employer and with the enviable equipment, having gotten his union card for that job specifically. He handed the foreman his ticket, expecting him to start talks about when to start and what to do next, but the foreman handed his ticket back to him and said, "I don't hire retards."

Not knowing what to do, shaken by what had just happened, he walked away.

"This is not uncommon. This is a very common thing I go through," he said before listing many other instances in his life when he was treated like garbage because of the shape of his head. At one job site, he was blamed for a major mistake by his coworkers, all their fingers pointing toward him, his cap covering the boat-like shape of his sagittal synostosis.

"There is nothing cosmetic about this surgery," he said. "I hate that term." In his very early forties, he has started to lose his vision. Blind spots have begun to cover parts of his eyes, shades of gray draping over the gelatinous curves of his eyes. Pressure has started to build up behind his eyes, enough pressure to pull him out of bed in the early morning to relieve it by sitting or standing upright. "There's nothing cosmetic about this."

"I've never shelled up. Like some people do. They self-exclude themselves. I've never done that," he said—the pride in his voice came out in deep, forceful words of confidence.

This prideful attitude, attached firmly to his feeling of otherness, became a part of him, like thick mesh weaving together at points and pulling apart at others, leaving gaps between the fabric strands that hold everything together. Someone must have the experience of being the other for long periods of time to grasp the significance of the words "This is not uncommon. This is a very common thing I go through." One's being, physical or emotional, worrying about what others see, hiding what makes him different, shaking with anticipation of a glance or long stare toward his head, becomes a foreigner to his own mind. If there was one time, maybe before the girl spoke in front of the classroom, that this person felt normal in the eyes of others, that feeling of normalcy, rattled loose by the continued glances toward what others see as an abnormality, it has drifted away like a paper lantern set on the water and destined to be crushed by the waves of the sea and only return to the shore in scattered, torn pieces, if it returns at all.

"These are battles I've fought all my life," he said.

* * *

Three months later, twelve hours before Cameron's surgery, the prescreening had been done. And something else has happened. Within the few days leading up to Cameron's surgery, the symptoms that other doctors had told the Pendletons to wait for have arrived. Like a strong flu in the night that comes on fast and strong, Cameron's head began to pound after he was running around and playing with his brothers, he stopped eating because he could not stand the pain in his head and the pain brought on by nausea, and his stomach woke in him in the night over the previous five or six weeks, whimpers and moans floating from his room to his parents, and all of this changed Shawn's mind for good. The ICP tests did not work. Shawn was the more reticent of the two, the one who worried that they might be opening their son's head for all the wrong reasons or for just shades of the right reason, but the symptoms that finally woke his son, the cries in the night that not only came from the pounding between the bony walls of his head but also from the soft, warm insides of his gut, and Dr. Staffenberg's words pulled Shawn away from any of those hang-ups about the surgery:

> One of the really interesting things about craniosynostosis is that there is something very organic about it that is not necessarily purely biochemistry. We're not talking about chemical reactions; we're talking about physical changes that may be visible in a baby, that may be harmful to the brain, that may have implications as the baby grows as far as not only their psychosocial development, their physical appearance, their self-esteem, but even their physical performance, you know? You know, we don't want to treat a baby who because of the original problem or because of the surgery now has limitations on their activity. Nothing makes me happier than being able to tell the parent that after the surgery's done the baby can do whatever they want to. I actually

got in trouble with mother and father once because I said, "Yeah, they can do whatever they want." So the way I say it now is, "They can do whatever you feel like letting them do." You don't want them to play football, they don't have to, but if you want them to play football and rugby, I want them to be able to do it. We've done the surgery in a way that will give us the best chance of having that. If your baby wants to grow up and shave his head and be on the swim team, then we're going to make a scar that will allow him to do that. I don't want to have a baby have a haircut a certain way or to wear their hair a certain way when they're older because of a bad scar. I want— I'm a plastic surgeon. I'm supposed to make that basically go away. The scar is permanent. It's always there, but I want it to be something that you have to show another person for them to notice.

So with craniosynostosis, so if we're talking about just simple things, sutures, and we're talking about the growth of the skull being impaired somehow, you know, the physical sort of conversation of what's going on is something that parents can get. And one of the most important things for them to understand, I think, from the beginning is that the skull itself does not have the innate programming to grow. The skull is passive. The only reason that the skull grows is because the brain is growing under it, so the brain is really dictating the shape of our head. The brain is dictating even how our face grows and what happens in craniosynostosis is that because one or more of the sutures have fused prematurely the skull is now dictating to the brain how it should grow. So it's now the reverse. The brain is being taken hostage by the skull, and so what we want to do, then, is release the hostage and allow the brain to resume normal control of the growth of the skull and the face. And that then brings us to another point, and we can get back to this, the timing of these operations. There was a time not too long ago that people were appalled that we would be talking about doing an operation, like any of these, on babies, and why not wait until they're fully grown? And actually, it was the unit here at NYU that started promoting sort of operation on babies because we knew from other kinds of pediatric surgery that babies could undergo anesthesia and things like that, but we were able to sort of stop all of the potentially bad things from developing, blindness or brain damage from the craniosynostosis. This is what happens when it's left alone to run its course and it's not intervened. It's a little bit like leaving a diabetic without treatment with insulin until they require an amputation. Well, if we'd managed their diabetes better, maybe we could prevent that from happening, so for the successful treatment of craniosynostosis we want to put the control of growth back where it should be so it makes sense that we're doing it on a baby before it goes really out of hand. We see babies that have bad craniosynostosis, when left alone, we actually will start to see changes in the shape of the face—asymmetries of the face, movement of the eye sockets, if it's left alone. And yet, if we operate early and remove that effect, then we can prevent all those bad things from happening. We left him and did these operations at sixteen to eighteen years old, then we'd be talking about more operations, another operation of treatment of the nose, another operation of treatment of the jaw, of the eyes. It doesn't make sense, so with each suture that gets closed we can actually predict a certain head shape and you know already, so if the suture down the middle of the forehead, the metopic suture, closes too early, we get that sort of triangular shape. If one of the coronal sutures down the side of the forehead closes too early, then we start getting sort of a lopsided appearance of the forehead. And the most common is when the sagittal closes down the middle the head becomes narrow and elongated. They each close from the bottom to the top like a zipper.

I had a ten-year-old boy that was never treated for it, and he said the other kids made fun of him because he has a forehead like a whale or a dolphin. Kids are cruel, but they know what they're talking about. They do cut to the chase.

In early June 2013 the Pendletons woke beneath the skyline of New York City, a far cry from their suburban home in Ohio. The East River ran wide and cold beyond the walls of NYC Medical and Dr. Staffenberg's office, where they had recently constructed a state-of-the-art surgical facility built specifically for children with cranial deformities and their parents. Large conference rooms, decorated with TVs and computers and comfy chairs, were built for larger, more open families who loved to hear everything together. Small, quaint, and intimate rooms were always to be used for small families, moms and dads who wanted a quiet consultation, and then operating rooms for the surgery.

Tara walked out of the apartment the Pendletons had rented on the Lower East Side into a cloudy, rainy day. The hovering clouds and raindrops comforted her, wrapping their wet arms around her. Later in the day, as the minutes and hours ticked slowly by, her son in surgery, she counted the drops on the window and watched them slowly streak downward like tears on a face. She didn't want a clear sky, the beautiful sun sitting in. She wanted the comfort of a rainy day and was happy when the clouds stayed with her until the night came.

Before surgery, the medical team asked if one parent would like to get into scrubs and follow them into the operating room until the cutting began. Tara, wanting to stay as close to her boy for as long as she could, volunteered and walked alongside some of the medical team into the room.

Cameron lay and waited. She watched the placement of IVs, the sticks of needles into the arms of her five-year-old boy who knew exactly what was going on, the fear that rushed through his eyes when they caught the worry in his mother's, the eyes that had done their best to stay strong over the last few years of his life, and the placement of the breather onto his mouth that filled the operating room with banana-scented anesthesia.

"I was prepared. I was being strong for him. I wanted to make him feel safe, but things happen very quickly, and my strength left me," she said.

The anesthesiologist told Cameron that he would just breathe in some bananas and then he would go to sleep. Sanitized rubber gloves moved around the boy like a magician's white gloves circling around an assistant lying on a table, moving smoothly and calmly without shaking—the hands moved so confidently from all their times there before—but this could not calm the mother who stood and watched her boy's body fight the anesthesia.

"It was so sad and so scary to see them strap the mask on and watch his body fight the anesthesia," Tara says. And even though the anesthesiologist said that the brawl between the brain and the body was normal—Tara knew that although the fighting between the brain and body was normal—putting the body under was not, and when the anesthesiologist placed her hand on Tara's back and told her she did good there was nothing in Tara's mind that could have kept her from falling into that dark place surrounded by her imagination saying that would be the last time she saw her son take in a breath.

"You did good, but it's time for you to join your husband," the anesthesiologist said to Tara.

While Tara's body walked out the door, escorted by the gentle hand of the anesthesiologist, her mind ran back to Cameron, grabbed him, and carried him out of there in her arms—that's all she wanted, to take him away and run, run, run away out into the rainy streets of New York City. But she made the eight to ten steps to the elevator. Her knees weakened. Her body shook. Several people stood around her in the elevator. Their breathing pumped the air around her thick and heavy. She was trapped in the elevator with all the fears of the last five years. They hit her like punches from a prizefighter, and all she could see was her son fall asleep and in that dark place she saw her son's last breath on this earth. Her fears punched and punched again, the fear of too much blood loss or a cut into the brain or another mistake, and she wished she had never stepped foot into the operating room, as she had to relive the movement of the rubber gloves, the placing of the IVs, the smell of bananas, and the last breath she saw her son take for the many long hours before Dr. Weiner came out and told her that Cameron's skull had been removed and that he was doing fine.

* * *

Tara talks into the microphone, her last recording of nine, three weeks post-op. Her boys play in the background, Cameron screaming among his brothers. Then her five-year-old boy joins her, his voice tiny as he is not sure what he is doing talking into a digital recorder in his hand. Tara giggles a bit. She asks him quietly to repeat what he asked her the day before, less than three weeks from the operating room. His voice, like the sound of an angel, speaks, this time confident in the sound of his words.

"Mommy, do you remember my headaches from yesterday before yesterday? Where'd they go?" he asks.

"Yes, I remember them," she answers.

He holds back for a second as if holding a punch line for a joke.

"They're gone, Mommy," he says. His voice is as cute as any little boy's voice could be—innocence laced with bravery. "I love my superhero scar."

* * *

After thirty-eight years, I do too, Cameron. I do too.

* * *

Release.

Bibliography

Agrawal, K., and S. Agrawal. "Tissue Regeneration During Tissue Expansion and Choosing an Expander." *Indian Journal of Plastic Surgery* 45.1 (2012): 7–15. Print and Web.

Bartlett, Scott, M.D. "Lambdoid Craniosynostosis: When a Flat Head Is Cause for Concern." The Children's Hospital of Philadelphia. 2012. Web.

Bhattacharya, Surajit. "Dr. Paul Tessier." *Indian Journal of Plastic Surgery* 41.2 (2008): 244–245.

Boyadjiev, Simeon A. "Genetic Analysis of Non-syndromic Craniosynostosis." *Ordodontics and Craniofacial Research* 10 (2007): 129–137.

Brown, Lesley, RN, and Mark R. Proctor. "Endoscopically Assisted Correction of Sagittal Craniosynostosis." *AORN Journal* 93.5 (2011): 582.

Burke, Edmund C., M.D. "Pediatric History: Abraham Jacobi, M.D.: The Man and His Legacy." *Pediatrics* 101.2 (1998): 309–312.

Chang, Anna, B.S., Eleonora M. Lad, M.D., Ph.D., and Shivanand P. Lad, M.D., Ph.D. "Hippocrates' Influence on the Origins of Neurosurgery." *Neurosurgical Focus* 23.1 (2007): E9. Print and Web.

Christiansen, Dorte M., Ask Elklit, and Miranda Olff. "Parents Bereaved by Infant Death: PTSD Symptoms Up to 18 Years After the Loss." *Journal of General Hospital Psychology*, 2013.

Clark, Kim, and Wes Clark. Personal Interview. 13 May 2013.

Claymen, M.A., G.J. Murad, M.H. Steele, and D.W. Pincus. "History of Craniosynostosis Surgery and the Evolution of Minimally Invasive Endoscopic Techniques: The University of Florida Experience." *Annals of Plastic Surgery* 58.3 (2007): 285–287.

The Cleveland Clinic Foundation. "Birth Defects." Cleveland Clinic Children's Hospital. 1 Sept. 2012. Web.

Cornelius, Carl-Peter. "Midface Coronal Approach." *AO Foundation.* 2009. Web. 9 Sept. 2013. Print.

Darnell, Laurie, and Joe Darnell. Personal Interview. 16 Jan. 2013.

Davidson, Shelby. Personal Interview. 20 March 2013.

DeVooght, Aimee. Personal Interview. 5 May 2013.

Dornelles, Rodrigo, Vera Cardim, and Nivaldo Alonso. "Skull Expansion by Spring-Mediated Bone Regeneration." *Acta Cirúrgica Brasileira* 25.2 (2010): 169–175.

Ehadi, Ali M., M.D., et al. "The Journey of Discovering Skull Base Anatomy in Ancient Egypt and the Special Influence of Alexandria." *Journal of Neurosurgical Focus* 33.2 (2012).

Ehmann, Summer, and Ryan Ehmann. Personal Interview. 10 Oct. 2012.

Engel, M. "Surgical Outcome After Using a Modified Technique of the Pi-Procedure for Posterior Sagittal Suture Closure."

Journal of Cranio-Maxillo-Facial Surgery 40 (2012): 363–368.

Ettus, Samantha. *The Experts' Guide to the Baby Years: 100 Things Every Parent Should Know.* New York: Random House, 2011.

Evoluciana. "Sima de los Huesos: The Largest Depository of Hominid Fossils Ever Discovered." Evoluciana.org. 10 Nov. 2013. Web.

Fearon, Jeffrey, M.D. Personal Interview. 2 May 2013.

Frassanito, Paolo, and Concezio Di Rocco. "Depicting Cranial Sutures: A Travel into the History." *Journal of Children's Nervous System*, 16 Dec. 2010. Web.

Goodrich, J.T., O. Tepper, and David Staffenberg. "Craniosynostosis: Posterior Two-third Cranial Vault Reconstruction Using Bioresorbable Plates and a PDS Suture Lattice in Sagittal and Lambdoid Synostosis." *Childs Nervous System* 28.9 (2012): 1399–1406.

Gracia, Ana, Juan Luis Arsuaga, Ignacio Martinez, Carlos Lorenzo, José Miguel Carretero, José Maria Bermúdez de Castro, and Eudad Carbonell. "Craniosynostosis in the Middle Pleistocene Human Cranium 14 from the Sima de los Huesos, Atapuerca, Spain." *Cranial Proceedings of the National Academy of Sciences* 106.16 (2008).

Grova, M., D.D. Lo, D. Montoro, J.S. Hyun, M.T. Chung, D.C. Wan, and M.T. Longaker. "Models of Cranial Suture Biology." *Journal of Craniofacial Surgery* 23.7 (2012).

Hajime, Arai, et al. "Craniosynostosis. Problems in Cranial Reconstruction Surgery in Patients with Craniosynostosis. Problems Related to Metallic Microplates and Excessive Tension upon Scalp Closure." *Nervous System in Children* 25.1 (2000): 33–37.

Hewitt, Jamie, and Stephen Hewitt. Personal Interview. 7 Jan. 2013.

Howard, Robyn, and Tommy Howard. Personal Interview. 17 March 2013.

Jane, John A., M.D. "Surgery for Craniosynostosis." Ed. Brian H Kopell, M.D. *Medscape.* Updated 17 Jan. 2014. Web.

Jeffreys, Nicole, M.D. Personal Interview. 31 Jan. 2014.

Jimenez, David F., and Constance M. Barone. "Endoscopic Technique for Sagittal Synostosis." *Childs Nervous System* Special Annual Issue, August 2012.

Johnstun, Bonnie, and Doyle Johnstun. Personal Interview. 10 Dec. 2013.

Karp, Harvey, M.D. *The Happiest Baby on the Block.* New York: Random House, 2008. Lee, Hui Qing, J.M. Hutson, A.C. Wray, P.A. Lo, D.K. Chong, A.D. Holmes, and A.L. Greensmith. "Changing Epidemiology of Nonsyndromic Craniosynostosis and Revisiting the Risk Factors." *Journal of Craniofacial Surgery* 23.5 (2012): 1245–1251.

Liu, Y., N. Kadlub, Freitas R. da Silva, J.A. Persing, C. Duncan, and J.H. Shin. "The Misdiagnosis of Craniosynostosis as Deformational Plagiocephaly." *Journal of Craniofacial Surgery* 19.1 (2008): 132–136.

Magge, Sheela N. "Long-term Neuropsychological Effects of Sagittal Synostosis on Child Development." *Journal of Craniofacial Surgery* 13.1 (2002): 1049–2275.

Maher, Cormac O., Steven R. Buchman, Edward O'Hara, and Aaron A. Cohen-Gadol. "Harvey Cushing's Experience with Cranial Deformity." *Neurosurgical Focus* 29.6 (2010): E6.

March of Dimes. "Birth Defects." March of Dimes. 1 Oct. 2011. Web.

McCarthy, Joseph G., Scot B. Glasberg, Court B. Cutting, Fred J. Epstein, Barry H. Grayson, Gregg Ruff, Charles H. Thorne, Jeffrey Wisoff, and Barry M. Zide. "Twenty-Year Experience with Early Surgery for Craniosynostosis: I. Isolated Craniofacial Synostosis—Results and Unsolved Problems." *Plastic and Reconstructive Surgery* 96.2 (1995): 212–283.

McFarland, Jennifer. Personal Interview. 3 May 2013.

Mehrara, Babak J., M.D. and Michael T. Longaker, M.D. "New Developments in Craniofacial Surgery Research." *Cleft Palate–Craniofacial Journal* 36, 37 (2000).

Mehta, Vivek A., C. Bettegowda, G.I. Jallo, and E.S. Ahn. "The Evolution of Surgical Management for Craniosynostosis." *Neurosurgical Focus* 29.6 (2010): E5.

Missios, Symeon, M.D. "Hippocrates, Galen, and the Uses of Trepanation in the Ancient Classical World." *Neurosurgical Focus* 23.1 (2007): E11.

Mowry, Bernice D. "Post-Traumatic Stress Disorder (PTSD) in Parents: Is This a Significant Problem?" Ed. Elizabeth Ahmann and Deborah Dokken. *Pediatric Nursing*, 5 May 2013. Web.

Nguyen, C., T. Hernandez-Boussard, R.K. Khosla, and C.M. Curtin. "A National Study on Craniosynostosis Surgical Repair." *Cleft Palate–Craniofacial Journal*, 2012.

Otto, Adolph Wilhelm. *A Compendium of Human & Comparative Pathological Anatomy*. London: B. Fellowes, 1831.

Pendleton, Tara, and Shawn Pendleton. Personal Interview. 5 Aug. 2013.

Podda, Silvio, M.D. "Craniosynostosis Management." *Medscape*. Updated 11 Nov. 2013. Web.

Rhoades, Camille, and Dustin Rhoades. Personal Interview. 13 Jan. 2013.

Shillito, John, Jr., and Donald D. Matson. "Craniosynostosis: A Review of 519 Surgical Patients." *Pediatrics* 41.4 (1968): 829–853.

Shultz, Myron. "Rudolf Virchow." *Emerging Infectious Diseases* 14.9 (2008): 1480–1481.

Smart, J.M., Jr., R.R. Reid, D.J. Singh, and S.P. Bartlett. "True Lambdoid Craniosynostosis: Long-Term Results of Surgical and Conservative Therapy." *Plastic Reconstructive Surgery* 120.4 (2007): 993–1003.

Staffenberg, David, M.D. Personal Interview. 7 Jan. 2013.

Taub, Peter J., and Joshua A. Lampert, M.D. "Pediatric Craniofacial Surgery: A Review for the Multidisciplinary Team." *Cleft Palate–Craniofacial Journal* 48.6 (2011): 670–683.

UNESCO. "Archaeological Site of Atapuerca." UNESCO. 2000. Web.

The U.S. National Library of Medicine. "Fetal Development." *Medline Plus*. 1 Oct. 2011. Web.

The U.S. National Library of Medicine. "Intercranial Pressure Monitoring." *Medline Plus*. 1 Oct. 2013. Web.

van der Meulen, Jacques. "Metopic Synostosis." *Childs Nervous System* 28 (2012): 1359–1367.

Velardi, F., A. Di Chirico, and C. Di Rocco. "Blood Salvage in Craniosynostosis Surgery." *Childs Nervous System* 15 (1999): 695–710.

Vesalius, Andreas. *On the Fabric of the Human Body*. Ed. Daniel Garrison, Daniel Malcolm Hast, and Northwestern University. Northwestern University. 2003. Web.

Walker, Marion, M.D. Personal Interview. 8 Oct. 2013.

Wan, Derrick, et al. "Craniofacial Surgery, from Past Pioneers to Future Promise." *Maxillofacial Oral Surgery* 8.4 (2009): 348–356.

Warren, Stephen M., M.D., Benjamin Walder, DDS, Wojciech Dec, M.D., Michael T. Longaker, M.D., and Kang Ting, DMD, DMSc. "Confocal Laser Scanning Microscopic Analysis of Collagen Scaffolding Patterns in Cranial Sutures." *Journal of Craniofacial Surgery* 19.1 (2008): 198–203.

Wexler, Andrew, and Leslie Cahan. "The Venetian Blind Technique: Modification of the Pi Procedure for the Surgical Correction of Sagittal Synostosis." *Journal of Craniofacial Surgery* 23.7 (2012): 2047–2048.

Zöllner, Alexander M. "Growing Skin: Tissue Expansion in Pediatric Forehead Reconstruction." *Biomechanics and Modeling in Mechanobiology* 11.6 (2012): 855–867.

Index

Numbers in **bold italics** indicate pages with photographs.